45 and

Pregnant

How I Conceived and Delivered

Naturally

LIZ ANGELES

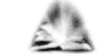

On the Inside Press
Beverly Hills, CA 90210

45 and Pregnant

How I Conceived and Delivered Naturally

Email the author - lovelizangeles@gmail.com

ISBN-13: 978-1-942707-08-0

Published by On the Inside Press
Beverly Hills, CA 90210
www.OntheInsidePress.com

Dedicated to my unforgettable mother

Suzan Valerie

who still works through me from the other side,

without whose love I could not have survived

and

to my greatest gift to the world I could provide,

Deja Isabella

My joy, my pride

ACKNOWLEDGMENTS

To Mario
For always being helpful, loving, supportive and devoted.
I am eternally grateful to you for waiting on me, hand and foot.
You are the best father conceivable.

To Annie
You have always been by my side and on my side,
with a warm and welcoming home away from home.
Your love and kindness, your help with my photos and your
beautiful photography are what make these memories so magical.

Thanks to Lori Dorman Photography for the cover photos.

CONTENTS

Act III - New Kid in Town

INTRODUCTION

If it's been said that a woman's chances of hitting the lottery are higher than her chance of getting married after 40, then the odds of starting a family are probably even lower. If that holds any truth, I might be one of the luckiest women alive. I found love at 44 and quickly got pregnant the traditional way — without even trying.

At 45 I delivered a bona fide love child with no drugs, incisions, complications or drama… all in a warm tub of water — in the privacy and comfort of my own home.

Honestly, if the biggest baby on the planet can do it (yes, that would be *me*), I'm sure millions more women can do it as well. Perhaps it's you who thinks it's too late to have children. Maybe it's your sister, your daughter, your aunt, your cousin or your best friend who wants to have a baby or a natural birth — or even a home birth over 40. Because my story has inspired so many women in my own circle of influence, I felt a calling to share my story with a larger audience.

If this book has made it into your hands, you are most likely from the camp that wants a natural birth. Perhaps you are on the fence and just being a good mom by doing your research. Perhaps you are considering in-vitro for the first or last time. For any or all of that, I applaud you. Education is key.

For those of you who want to hear first-hand from a woman who has been through it herself, I will explain why I wouldn't hesitate to make the same choices if I had to do it all over again.

I am not here to judge anyone for their beliefs or choices, because we are all unique with so many variables that form our lives and who we are. I am not an expert in motherhood, pregnancy, hospitals, home birth or children. As a health conscious person for most of my life, a massage therapist for 25 years and a yogi for 15 years, I would not consider myself an expert in health, wellness or even writing. Like you, I am just a woman who wants to look and feel my best, wants the best for my child, and wants to get through the day the best way I know how.

I had always believed I would never really grow up until I became a mother—to more than merely my own inner child. I was right. Now that I am a mother, I find I'm an even bigger work in progress with much growing ahead of me.

I have lived and learned from having been a well-loved child, a dedicated student, a stubborn bratty drama queen, a self-sufficient scrapper, a life-of-the-party girl, a serial monogamist, a motherless daughter and a compassionate healer. In my nearly half a century on Earth, emotionally, I have been all over the map. I have studied and explored. I have read as many self-help books as I have had problems, and along the way I have found stillness.

What I do strongly believe in is the law of attraction. I believe that our thoughts and feelings create our reality.

Through my studies and practices, I have come to believe that letting go of stress and worry is like taking down a wall that stands between you and your desires. Admittedly, that is a constant challenge. Trusting in fate is truly liberating. Trusting in your *own* strength is monumentally empowering.

Because there are three distinct parts to my story, I have taken artistic license and broken it down into three acts rather than chapters. I suppose I'm still an actress at heart, and—well, I'm just an all-around unconventional gal.

You may think I share a little too much information in this book, and I would be the first to agree. This is a *very* personal journey. If you find yourself bored in the first part of my story, feel free to skip ahead to ACT II – *Making Womb for a New Mom*, which is highly informative and provides details into my pregnancy over 40—yes, even as late as 45. I decided to share the information I collected that may help you with the many tough choices that lie ahead. I really do understand and empathize with the anxiety these decisions can create.

You might be one who enjoys reading intimate details of someone else's life. If your life is far more put together than mine was, ACT I—*Prelude to a Kid* may give you more confidence to question "If *she* can do this....*why can't I?*"

Because my experience could not have been more successful, I would like to continue carrying the torch for home birth. Nothing would make me happier than to know my story could inspire more women longing to become empowered with this type of birth experience.

This is not a "how to" book. It's just *my* story. I suppose it's a "how I" book. You may wonder why I go off on tangents about things that don't relate directly to my pregnancy or a natural birth. I am hoping to give you a broader scope about my life experiences that led me to make specific choices.

Take what you can use and ignore what does not work for you. We all have a unique experience. Things can't always go as planned, so honor what comes up and accept any outcome, as everything happens for a reason.

My greatest hope is that you find my journey enlightening, educational and above all, inspiring. At the very least, you may pick up some highly useful information and have a few good laughs along the way.

ACT I

Prelude to a Kid

The Predicament...
No Man = NO Baby

Finding love in this world can be a life-long pursuit, and even more difficult in Los Angeles. Trust me, I've been around the block again and again. I've been around the sun multiple times — for shall we say ... many moons? And suffice it to say, my moon has been in many places and that was clearly 'fruitless.'

Eventually, you either go on Match.com for the zillionth time, or throw your hands up in despair and hit the couch only to bury yourself in a cable coma. With beautiful people turning our heads around every corner, and in our instant gratification culture, it seems there is always something better on the horizon — greener grass in every pasture. Many have said the search for love in Los Angeles is futile and the only way to find a real gentleman is to simply move out of town.

As the girl whose own mother thought she was not "the settling down type," I have, regardless, been a hopeless romantic since puberty. As a serial monogamist with relationships that never lasted more than a year or two, always ending up single *again*, the prospect of finding my soul mate was growing increasingly unlikely as the years went on.

By 38, I was terribly depressed, living in Las Vegas, the very city in which I had hoped to never again reside. I was living with my very kind stepdad in the house he and my late mother had purchased together. I was still recovering from her death two years prior. She died the night before 9/11/2001. It was definitely a one-two punch that left me in a daze for a couple of years.

7

By the year 2003, I was recovering from a break-up with a man who had swept me off my feet. I gave up my beautiful rent-controlled apartment in Santa Monica—he had enthusiastically assured me we were heading to the altar. This was the same year I would lose my mother.

So by 2003 my life had been entirely gutted. When I moved back to Las Vegas, this ex-boyfriend in Santa Monica had already moved on and quickly impregnated a woman half my age. How cliché, right?

Not long after hearing that little nugget of ego-crushing information, I learned that Britney Spears was pregnant. I remember literally bursting into tears when I heard that news. Here she was, so young and successful and already starting a family, thereby "having it all" in my mind.

By comparison, at 38 I felt washed up. Here I was, living in the bedroom above the garage, in the far northwest corner of the Las Vegas Valley. I was miserable and thought my life couldn't be more pathetic.

In fact, it could be *much* worse than that. These days, with all my first-world problems, I count my blessings by remembering that 40% of the world's population will never know what it's like to have running water. How spoiled *are* we?

While in Vegas, I became obsessed with my goal of returning to Santa Monica. I am a true California girl. I was born in and raised in Healdsburg, a very small town in Northern California's wine country. I'm very grateful to have been raised in that environment—it's so wholesome and gorgeous. The saddest part of childhood is that we never understand gratitude or how good we have it.

I do know that I prefer the Southern California climate. In fact, I am now very committed to L.A. I love it so much I literally married it. Yes, folks, you heard it here first. I legally changed my last name to *Angeles* so I could officially use the name *Liz Angeles* in business. You probably assumed my parents were crazy or kooky—and yes, you would be right—but the buck stops here. There is a method to my madness. People remember my name. They could never remember the name *Wilmarth*, so it had to go. Read it out loud. Doesn't it feel like you are about to toss your cookies?

When I moved back to Vegas, still using my maiden name at 38, I thought it was high time for a new identity and a new name anyway. In contrast to *Wilmarth*, Liz *Angeles* just rolls of the tongue. Try it—you can even say it with your teeth clenched, while smiling!

When I was still living and working as a realtor in Santa Monica, I met a woman named Susan Jeffers, a prolific writer and well-known author of *Feel the Fear and Do it Anyway*. We were chatting and she asked me if I had kids. When I told her I wasn't sure what terrified me more—having them or not having them—she said, "Oh dear, you need to read my book," and immediately handed me a copy of *I'm OK, You're a* Brat!

Ms. Jeffers hit the nail on the head that day. That book completely changed my mentality and reckoning with whatever was in my destiny. I quickly realized I would be "OK" if I never had kids. However, I had always assumed that I would become a mother at some point. Although that "some point" I had always pictured at least five years down the road, and never in my *immediate* future.

I've never been "baby crazy" or gotten pregnant by accident, or even tried to get pregnant. I was always careful because I took that responsibility very seriously. I had never given a man an ultimatum or left a relationship because a boyfriend wasn't ready for kids, as many women do. That concept has always bewildered me.

9

By the time I turned 40, I had come to accept I would probably not have kids. The more stories I would see about child molestations or kindergarten hostages, the more terrorizing motherhood seemed and the less I felt I was destined to become a mother.

Top three reasons I assumed I was not equipped for motherhood:

1) I don't handle stress well

2) I hate loud noises

3) I require a lot of sleep to function.

Any mother would tell me, "Yep. It's probably not a good idea."

Finally, I decided if it were meant to happen, it would. I had no compulsion to adopt and never dreamt of tempting fate with the prospect of in-vitro fertilization.

Who knew if my eggs were even good? I assumed they were probably rotten by 40. How many women get pregnant naturally over 40? I read that the chances of getting pregnant naturally over 43 are about 1 to 2 percent.

Fortunately, I had always been a health nut, which began in my late teens. I even taught aerobics in the 80's at the height of Jane Fonda's fitness craze. I was a Physical Education major at UNLV with a minor in dance and was constantly either at the gym or in the dance studio.

Over a decade later, in my mid 30's, I was much less ambitious and then fell in love with yoga. At that age, I was finally ready to settle down, but I was still attracting toxic relationships. Since the right man for the job still hadn't appeared in my life, I would have to wait it out and hope for the best.

Perhaps my early obsession with health and fitness was an auspicious start that gave me a leg up, making the maintenance to stay in shape easier as I aged. *Perhaps* my chances were better than pregnancy statistics would predict. It was all yet to be determined.

A feng shui master did my numbers when I was 40 and he told me, "You will probably meet your soul mate around 42. But your soul mate probably won't want to marry." I said, "Yep, that sounds like my soul mate!" Later, still in my early 40's, a Venice Beach boardwalk palm reader (with a very thick Asian accent) told me, "You may have two or three chi-ren, but you have a lot of fears and a lot of worries, so you may have a more comfortable life if you don't have chi-ren." Amen! I knew he could not have been more accurate.

As most women do, I fantasized about a beautiful wedding with a gorgeous dress, but I also took a very realistic view of it. My parents were married four times each and didn't get it right until their final attempts. I didn't feel that marriage was something that should be rushed into. Call me crazy, but I had no problem jumping head first into love and monogamy time and time again. But committing for the rest of my life? Yikes!

Parental break-ups were so hard on me as a child, and my own break-ups were devastating enough, with or without cohabitation. It seemed to me that marriage was perhaps obsolete, or at the very least, anti-climactic. It seems like a wedding is often the "kiss of death," and so humiliating when marriages don't last. I didn't want to become another Elizabeth Taylor or Kim Kardashian, lives littered with the mayhem of multiple divorces.

Marriage seems a daunting and arduous chore, seen as a failure if it doesn't last, when people change and grow apart over years together, especially when they marry young. How can anyone know for sure they want to be with someone until they die?

One of my favorite comedians, Aziz Ansari, does a bit about how creepy a proposal is. It goes something like this: "Imagine the guy is all infatuated with you, and says, 'You know how we've been hanging out a lot and getting along really well? I want to do that until you're dead!'" I can see how he would think that might seem creepy.

My hairdresser told me that many women confess if they had to do the wedding again, they would keep it small and save the money for a home or something more long lasting.

Bill Murray publicly declared his philosophy, "If you use your wedding money traveling the world with someone, and *if* you still want to be together after that, *then* get married." That makes sense to me.

Wedding days are so stressful and the bride almost never even has a chance to enjoy it. I actually structured my life specifically to *avoid* stress because it is the number one cause of illness and disease. I still practice massage after 25 years because I am doing the best thing I can think to do by relieving people of that deadly stress.

You would think someone who is naturally nurturing would be the ideal candidate to become a mother. You would *think...* but finding the right partner is the prerequisite and doing it alone just didn't appeal to me.

While living in Las Vegas, I was giving a massage at the Four Seasons Hotel and the client asked me about my background and childhood. I explained that I grew up between two brothers and have had two half sisters, two half brothers, two stepsisters, and one stepbrother. My dad had 7 children (that we know of) from 4 different women. In the course of one year in the early 60's, he actually had three women pregnant. Ah, the time of free love. My half sister was born just 8 days after me, and her brother was born just a few months before my older brother.

Clearly, everyone would agree that my dad's weakness was loving women too much. But it *was* the 60's and he was in his 20's. He was still a good dad who always showed up, constantly told us he was proud of us and that he loved us. That's big. Many people never have that. I tend to focus on the good in people – to my detriment? Perhaps at times, but I would go crazy if I didn't. I feel very blessed to have had very loving, supportive parents.

This client responded with, "Oh my God! Do the world a favor and don't have kids!" When I asked, "Why not?" He answered, "You don't need to perpetuate that level of dysfunction!" I laughed it off, but for years after I wondered if maybe he was blessed with foresight.

Still, we all want to leave this world knowing we did some good, and perhaps left behind something of great value, someone or something that really matters; a legacy.

As I was getting older, assuming my eggs were rotten and my chance to bear children had passed, I knew I had to do something to feel fulfilled. It felt increasingly imperative to find a way to walk through the rest of my life without wondering if my existence was a total waste of space.

So it was during my most financially lucrative (and most lonely) years in Vegas that I became very productive with creativity by painting. I felt that was something I could leave behind when I kicked the bucket. My paintings were like my babies. *They* would be my legacy. My passion is creating a piece with color, theme and style that pulls the whole room together.

I also spent those years in Vegas from 2005 to 2007 as a sales rep helping my buddies grow their new company. We manufactured and sold an extremely popular and effective natural male enhancement supplement. We couldn't get the product made fast enough. It was constantly on back order.

Many men were in awe of its power. My doctor even sold it to his patients. What I loved most about selling it was hearing the stories from rather elderly couples about their rekindled romance.

Sadly, the product was recalled because of alleged adulteration and would be removed from the shelves of the 200 accounts I had personally opened across the country. After all my hard work, it was incredibly depressing to lose that revenue stream.

The upside? By 2007 I had sold enough to generate the funds necessary to relocate back to Santa Monica. I longed to live near the ocean breeze, where creativity is ubiquitous, yoga is on every corner, and health food is more accessible. Santa Monica is a far more progressive and spiritual community than the money-obsessed, sex-oriented, drug-driven, concrete faux jungle of Las Vegas. But to its credit, Vegas *is* making progress.

Going Back to Cali

Being single in L.A. can be brutal. Sure, there are hot guys everywhere—and even more hot girls, for that matter. Eye candy galore is here for you if you ever get the opportunity to move to Los Angeles.

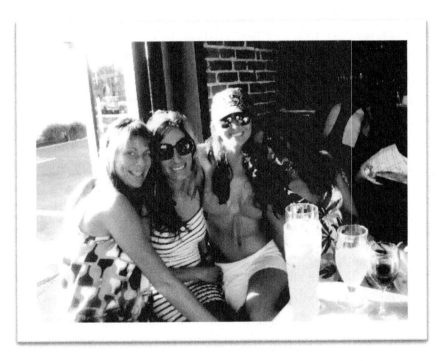

Caroline, Angela, Me, Stephanie, Venice 2009

Even in this huge dating pool, the 'pickins' can be slim for women over 40. I believe it's mostly because we've become hyper particular about the men we might choose to be our life partners. Actually, I believe we have a wider range of men who *are* interested. First, you have the men around your age range (who should be a good match if they aren't dating women half their age). Then you have the older, often retired or very successful men who see you as a young spring chicken — a nice perk.

Finally, you have the young men who *love* the women they see as MILFs. It seems to have become very fashionable for young men to date older women — probably because we don't usually want anything serious from the youngsters and we aren't afraid to ask them to hit the road when we are finished with them. They could be great for a steamy roll in the hay or even as mere sperm donors. They find us sexy, seasoned, wise and experienced. At least that's what *we* hear! I think what men find sexy is the same thing women find sexy; good old-fashioned confidence — that and a genuine smile. The two never go out of style.

As we age and let go of our insecurities, we become more of who we are and let go of what doesn't serve us. Perhaps you have noticed the ease on the face of a self-actualized person and their total lack of pretense. I believe it's their overall presence and purpose — it's what compels us to dig deeper. Outer beauty becomes quickly boring and uninteresting if there is no inner spark that stirs beneath the surface.

Think about it. If you look at yourself in the mirror, you aren't usually smiling or excited about something. Instead, you are judgmental and critical of yourself. That's never a good look on anyone's face. But let's say you have a conversation on the phone with a fun friend while you look in the mirror, you can see another side of yourself. *That's* your inner beauty. I have found people stay interesting by staying interested … in anything. That spark will light you up from the inside.

All the Single Ladies

Once back in Santa Monica, I was literally BLIZFUL. So much so, that I had that put on my license plate. It's easy to attract a man when you are out with your girlfriends, happy with your life and just beaming with joy.

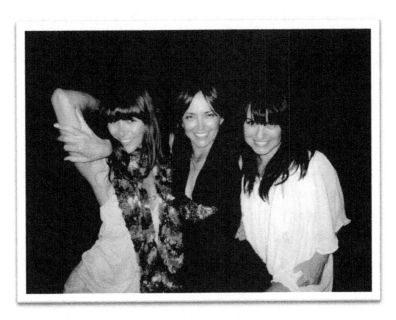

Malia, Me, Marla – Girls Night Out

Therefore, it wasn't long before I met a great guy who was a tall, dark and handsome attorney. He was just a bit younger than I was, but still not ready for commitment – at least not to me. It wasn't like I was dying to be a wife, as much as I just wanted a decent boyfriend. That relationship only lasted a few months and left me feeling rather hopeless once it was over. It took me over a year to recover from that, probably because it became more and more challenging to meet a man who I wanted to hang out with for an entire weekend, let alone the *rest of my life!*

Many of my male friends at that time were confused and baffled about why I was still single. I would always answer those remarks with the question, "Have you noticed all my other hot, amazing, talented, kind, fun-loving girlfriends? We are all perplexed!"

I would counter their question with another, "Let me ask you this: Do *you* know any great guys that would be a good match for me, that you would set me up with?" They always answer, "No, actually I don't." Any guy will even tell you that most guys are idiots, pigs, douche bags, etc. I still have hope for men but it does seem all the best ones get scooped up quickly.

I saw a great post on Facebook about how low-lying fruit is easier to pick and the truly delicious ripe ones up top are harder to reach. It makes sense that it applies to women as well. We all just want a smart guy who is fun, clean, decent looking, healthy, financially responsible and hopefully funny. Well, I want a lot more than that in a man, but that's another story entirely.

What changed everything was probably my diligence in believing in LOVE.

I already had years of experience with practicing the law of attraction. Therefore I had honed the list of the qualities I sought in my ideal man, aptly titled, "Liz's Dreamboat." Still, I was very lonely.

Because my friends and I are always working on our dreams and aspirations, I joined in a "prosperity circle" for women at my buddy Annie's place. We took turns describing what we wanted for our lives so the rest of us could help it manifest with the group intention—the power in our numbers.

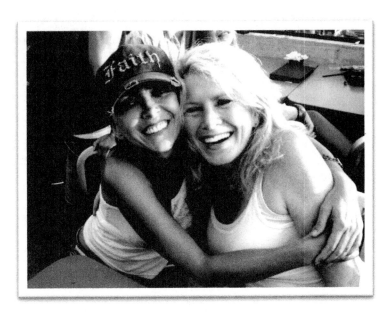

With my BFF Annie Flatley - Summer 2009

Each woman described their wish for this or that career, fame, home, or amount of money they wanted to attract. When it was my turn, my wish wasn't for fame or money.

What I had always wanted deep down

was to experience the love of a child

that only a mother knows.

Since I was 44 and that time had clearly passed, I explained what I *most* wanted was a *famous love* that people talked about, remembered, and aspired to have. I never had anything close to that, but before I was pushing up daisies, I wanted it more than *anything* else.

This meeting happened in late February of 2009. By the end of the summer, I had officially put my quest for love on the back burner and put my own creative goals and aspirations on the front burner. What happened next is what I can describe as nothing less than a divine intervention.

Divine Intervention

One beautiful Sunday afternoon, *precisely* six months later, I was at Annie's bungalow in Venice and we were excited about our new business venture to decorate homes on a modest budget, creating magic with comfort and tranquility in mind. We called it *L.A. Homegirlz.*

While we were researching lighting stores and talking about finding a handyman to help us, I received a phone call from a woman named Alexia who told me she had the best massage she has ever had from *me.* She was certain she knew me, but I was certain I didn't know *her.* She told me she had a friend who was unable to leave his house due to a bad back and asked if I could help. A few minutes later he called me. His name was Mario.

Mario proceeded to tell me about how he threw his back out lifting a fireplace. I learned he was an out-of-work general contractor on the verge of getting evicted due to the shenanigans of his teenage daughters. Mario told me about his back and that he had only been able to walk from the couch to his bed for the last month, and could no longer stand it. He asked if I could come over that afternoon.

I had just come from yoga and told him I needed to bike home to shower and then I could go. He then says, "I don't care what you smell like. I just want your hands on my body." Ahem... What? Did he really just say that? Yes, he did. I think I may have actually blushed. Had he even seen a picture of me from my website? No. He was just that desperate for healing.

I did have a weakness for those hot-blooded Latin men. He was Colombian and Spanish. He sounded cute, so I thought to dress cute *just in case!* I remember very clearly questioning my own motives, "Come on Liz, why would you ever want to get involved with someone who has sole custody of teenage girls and is out of work anyway?"

When I showed up at his apartment in Westwood, his brother came down to carry my massage table upstairs. "Wow," I thought to myself as I walked up the stairs, "If this is Sergio, I can't wait to meet *Mario!*" When I walked in the door, the man sitting on the couch looked just like Sergio but had very long hair pulled back in a loose braid. He wore nothing but a sexy pair of eyeglasses, and a pair of loose-fitting basketball shorts.

When I first saw Mario, all I remember thinking was, "Wow, I get to massage *this* guy? Yummy!" I set up my table and proceeded to work on his body. Immediately, the sparks began to fly. This *never* happens. On his forearms, (one of my favorite male body parts) were twin pieces of a statue that his anthropologist uncle had found in Colombia. He was revered for it because it was a missing link in their culture. It was called *Doble Yo* meaning "Double Me," which is fitting, since Mario is a Gemini. His daughters' names and birthdays were inscribed within the statues, camouflaged in a hieroglyphic-style font.

On his left shoulder was a beautiful tattoo of his favorite person on the planet, his mother. This was a very good sign. My previous boyfriend had little or no respect for his mother. Men who don't respect their mothers don't tend to respect women as easily. Mario tells me he learned *everything* from his mother and that his father died miserably, riddled with cancer.

I noticed Mario was extremely passionate and a very interesting conversationalist. At this point I assumed I was older than him because he looked like he was in his mid 30's. I was shocked to find out he was 46—refreshingly older than me. He was equally shocked to find out I was 44. I had always wanted to meet an older soul in a younger shell or at least someone who

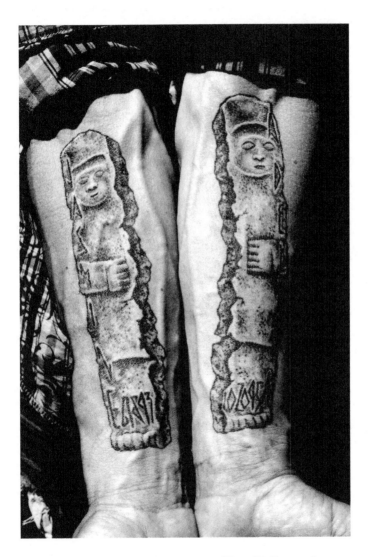

Doble Yo by ZULU Tattoo, West Hollywood

kept himself in good shape. He was tan, lean and light (how I like my men).

23

His 16-year-old daughter Jasmine walked by the room where I was setting up and looked me up and down, as if I were a threat to her territory. I felt a familiar jolt, like I knew her from a past life. I loved the way he addressed her, as simply *Babydoll* or *Beautiful*. I thought that would be so nice to hear that from your dad all the time. My dad only called me *Sis* because I was the middle child and only girl.

Mario and I talked during the entire massage and spilled our souls to each other quickly. When I told him about the home-decorating business Annie and I were starting, he was quick to offer up his services without my having to ask.

After the massage, he made a comment about my feet. I admitted that every man with a foot fetish goes crazy over them. His smile said it all. I knew I had him. I gave him my card. My name gave him a chuckle. He gave me a generous tip for someone who had been out of work for several months.

Suddenly, he seemed to be walking around with no problem. He wasn't strong enough to help me carry my table downstairs, but was eager to accompany me as I returned to my car.

I don't know if it was the sparks flying that gave him the energy to make the trip, or if I healed him to the point he could move around more easily, but as I was leaving he definitely looked like a new man. Standing there in the middle of the street in his shorts and bare feet, with his long hair blowing in the ocean breeze, wearing the biggest, most beautiful smile you have ever seen, Mario watched me drive away.

I could tell when I was leaving that it was *on*. I would definitely be seeing him again. I also knew I needed to play it cool because I did *not* want to get emotionally involved with him. I was determined to stay focused on my new business venture and would not let any man come between me and my dream. But I also *knew* I needed to touch him again.

The big mystery: months later, I finally met Alexia, the woman who referred me to massage Mario. She said, "No, I've never met you." I knew that. To this day, we still have *no* idea how she got my card, or how I was ultimately led to Mario. There may be no better way to explain it other than simply 'divine intervention.'

The Romance

The next day I received a voice mail from Mario saying he was so happy to meet me, that he really appreciated my massage, and that he would love to work out a trade with me. At the time, I was living in Venice because I wanted to live around more artists. That night I went out with my girlfriends Marla and Malia to *The Brig* in Venice. I was giddy because Mario kept texting me.

I was probably glowing when I unexpectedly ran into my ex-boyfriend. For the first time, I was happy to see him. Men always seem so quick to replace women after a break up. It felt good to be excited about someone new, finally — after a year and a half of lonely nights.

Like most women, I could easily pick up a man if I really needed one. Finding someone whose company I enjoy on a regular basis is another challenge altogether.

During Mario's next massage, I remember saying how nice it was to massage a man with long hair because I like to massage the scalp and gently pull the hair, as it is so relaxing. When he said, "It would be fun to get our hair tangled up together," I assumed he must not be attached to another woman.

This is when I knew it was really *on*. But I was still unsure about this eccentric looking, longhaired, earring-adorned, broke contractor with *teenagers*, who's still hobbling around with a cane.

The next time I saw Mario, when he walked in the door, we suddenly fell into an embrace. No words were spoken. We just stood there holding each other for what seemed like several minutes, but what was probably only one or two. That's a long time to be holding someone when we'd had no obvious mention of any sort of pending date or mutual attraction.

He quickly went to work as my new handyman in my apartment. After he finished, I asked him if he would mind rubbing my shoulders for a couple of minutes. Naturally, he was delighted. This shoulder rub was much needed and coming from him, felt *amazing*! However, it didn't last long before it happened.

We finally kissed. That kiss was utterly ridiculous, in the most epic way possible. He was almost *too* into it, if that's possible. He didn't waste any time professing his feelings for me. What came out of his mouth made me question his sanity. "I would kill for you. I would die for you. I would build you an empire."

Part of me thought this guy is completely cracked! But the hopeless romantic in me *loved* it. Almost immediately after he left, I called my girlfriends Angela and Carolyn to tell them about our afternoon tryst. For a moment there is silence on the other end. Carolyn suddenly blurted, "Let him build you an empire. We all need a place to stay!" We roared with laughter.

Mario left me with a fluttering heart beating a mile a minute. He had to return to his kids and I had a very hot date that night to watch the fireworks at the Santa Monica Pier for its 100-year anniversary. I had been looking forward to this date, but once we finally got together, I found myself thinking about Mario the entire time. This is when I *knew* I was in serious trouble.

A Motherless Daughter

On that night, I was thinking of my late mother, who passed away the night before 9-11. It was the eve of the anniversary of her death. I was watching the fireworks over the pier thinking how much she would love them.

I felt her energy in my life, still organizing and orchestrating on my behalf. Things seemed to be going well for me, and I was finally feeling at peace with the lack of her presence in my life.

My mom and I were very close. We were best friends, like sisters, and I can recall fewer than a dozen fights with her in my entire life. I always thought she could do no wrong and she was my biggest fan. We were grateful to have such a healthy friendship, especially when many mother-daughter relationships are so often contentious. Our relationship was one to be envied. She's the one in my family who would always visit me in Los Angeles. She's the one I would visit for family holidays or run to when I was troubled or heartbroken.

My mother Suzan loved Las Vegas and worked in casinos since I was 10 years old. She began in the 1970's downtown at the Union Plaza, and ended her career with the opening of the Venetian. It was her dream job. She was a Table Games Supervisor, or 'pit boss.'

She had three children by the time she was 22, so she was a young, fun-loving, productive and busy mom. Mom had always looked ten years younger than she was. When anyone would meet her, they were shocked that she could have a daughter my age.

I was especially hard hit when I learned this vibrant loving woman had multiple myeloma and was told she had two to five years left to live.

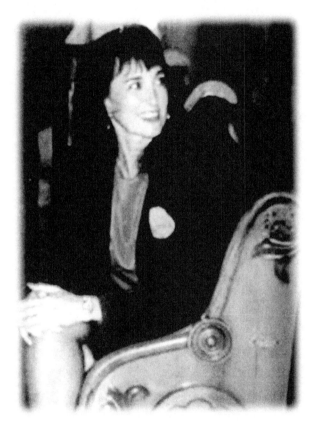

My Mom Suzan, 1990 Age 45

Bone marrow cancer is especially painful and miserable. After five nauseating months of chemotherapy, they sent her home with balloons and celebrated that they had 'rid her body of any trace of cancer.' She was *thrilled* to return to her job.

As she was getting ready for work, she realized she was too weak to go in. The chemo had taken such a toll, that by the time they rid her body of cancer, the rest of her organs shut down and she was then informed there was nothing more they could do for her. She would ride out the rest of her life in a hospice—only to die a slow, miserable and painful death.

Early on, I campaigned for her to try a holistic alternative, but she and my stepfather were sold on traditional western medicine. She couldn't bear to stomach my healthful alternatives and refused to drink my fresh vegetable juice, so I felt helpless and was forced to watch her slowly deteriorate over a 9-month period and die—regardless of the treatment. She didn't even make it one more year, let alone 'two to five.'

This only made me question western medicine that much more.

I asked the doctor, "If chemotherapy doesn't help, and it ultimately killed my mother, why on Earth do you prescribe it?" All her doctor could tell me is that it's what they are taught and sold. It literally makes me sick when I think about it.

In the early phase of her illness, my research led me to two videos by Dr. Lorraine Day. *You Can't Improve on God* and *Cancer Doesn't Scare Me Anymore.* Lorraine Day is a doctor who was stricken with cancer and refused chemotherapy because of its effects she observed in her own practice. She knew it was prescribed because all doctors are sort of seduced and strong-armed to perpetuate the machine.

Instead, Dr. Day went the natural route and completely healed herself of a grapefruit-sized tumor in her chest with things like juicing and avoiding meat. She combined that with lots of meditation, positive visualization and prayer.

She claims the American Medical Association and the American Cancer Society are out for profit. I had always suspected this was the case, but it's a very different experience hearing it from an educated and experienced medical doctor.

I wished my mother had tried listening to me. She and my stepfather had been so proud and happy about the weight they lost on the Atkins diet, which largely consisted of meat consumption. I therefore couldn't help but wonder if that contributed to her demise.

Louise Hay's book *You Can Heal Your Life* will say that cancer of the bone stems from deep resentment. This made sense because my mother had raised three children with a man who had stepped outside of the relationship so much, that he had three other children born within just months of our births. We never even knew they existed until our late 20's when they wanted to meet our dad. Keeping secrets that big *must* make one sick, and it makes good sense that Mom would become a party girl and escape that level of pain.

Clearly, coming from a broken home would lead someone like me to therapy, but since I've never been able to afford it, I sought out a deeper understanding of myself through dozens of self-help books. In one called *In The Meantime* by Iyanla Vanzant, I remember the author making the point that

"While our mothers are pregnant,

we are marinating in her emotions."

This explained a lot to me. While my dad was out with *other women*, she must not have felt worthy, or that a man would ever be there for her. Vanzant also discusses how

"The event of our birth sets the blueprint for our psyche."

My father's absence at my birth may have led me to believe on some level that no man would be there for me either. Perhaps I expect them to let me down. It's always been the norm for me.

This might explain why I found myself single at 44 with no relationship lasting longer than two years—and why I needed to be sure I had a man truly worthy of fathering a child, who would be there for me and for my child—*prior* to taking that leap.

Perhaps my dad's absence during that time affected my attracting the wrong men. No matter how much men may love you, they still have their dark sides.

I always knew that if I ever got pregnant, I hoped to have a stress-free pregnancy, if at all possible. I also knew it would be wise to become financially independent *before* becoming pregnant. My life experience up to that point didn't give me much hope for *any* relationship surviving the many challenges of parenthood— let alone compatible cohabitation.

As a natural-born worrier, I asked my mom one day how she handled all the worries that accompany motherhood. She told me something that saves me almost every day when I feel myself going down that road. She said, "I learned very early on that there is no point in worrying until the time comes to worry. Then you just deal with what you have on your plate at the time." Genius.

The Courtship

Mario courted me the old fashioned way. It was refreshing not to feel rushed into sex. He took his time getting to know me. He would actually call me and ask me if I was free for a date. Men just don't do that anymore. They text you late at night and ask, "What are you up to?" The male gender seems to have grown that lazy. Perhaps it's a condition of American men. Mario is Colombian and was raised by a very strict Spaniard who taught him chivalry.

When he picked me up for our first date, I couldn't believe how clean and nice his car was. I assumed he had borrowed it from someone because I had only seen him in his beat up, old work truck. This car was unbelievably spotless inside and out.

My impression of him was abruptly altered. He is a complete clean freak in *certain* areas of his life. Honestly, watching him organize a cabinet or pantry to maximize space at high speed or vacuuming behind the couch and under the cushions are all things that should be videotaped and sold as 'porn for women.'

We had a remarkable first date. After we had drinks at the *World Café* in Santa Monica, we met three of my girlfriends at *Nikki's Beach* in Venice. They had each heard good things about him, so one by one, they each proceeded to give him a hug and a kiss on the lips. After kisses from three more beautiful women, he thought he had died and gone to heaven. He said he felt like he was 16 again.

I was preparing to take a trip to Washington DC for a trade show the next day, and he asked me if he could drive me to the airport. Who does that? Certainly no guy I had just begun to date, so he was quickly gaining points. It wasn't long before he swept me off my feet with those charms. He told me about how and why he got full custody of his daughters when they were 11 and 13. He also said he would have another child—that he loved the baby thing, diapers and all, describing it all as *"awesome!"*

In my mind, I'm thinking, "Awesome?" He was quickly fulfilling all of the requirements I desired in a relationship - just knowing he was open to having another child opened the door for him even more.

Still, he had teenagers and no job at the time, and *I* didn't make much money, so it wasn't like I had much hope of "marrying well," financially speaking. Then again, money had never been a prerequisite for a man in my life, by any means. I've known a lot of miserable people with plenty of money and even more who were spiritually and emotionally challenged.

While I was in DC, we spoke on the phone every night, and toward the end of my trip he offered to fly me home earlier so I could see him sooner. At that time, I had another job working for ABILITY magazine—for people with disabilities. That particular job constantly reminded me how lucky I was to be healthy and strong and have all of my working parts.

As I edited articles about people rising above serious hardships they are faced with, I was continually inspired and reminded that I should stop whining altogether. I encountered several stories about disabilities—often birth defects—reminding me that what a woman does or does not do while she is pregnant can dramatically affect her child's entire life, as well as the mother's life.

After the trade show in DC, my boss took us to the White House. We had just missed seeing President Obama on the lawn because we were a little *too late*. (Bad timing—the story of my life).

When I spoke to the armed guard at the White House gate about the magazine, he started talking to me about his daughter with autism and—perhaps as he was thinking about his struggles with her affliction—he began to cry. It's odd to see a big, burly armed guard with tears in his eyes, but still very humanizing. It made me seriously question things that may lead to autism.

The guard offered to give me a personal tour of the White House the next day. A lifetime opportunity, right? Instead of doing that, I took Mario up on his offer and came home early so we could be together. It *must* have been *love*.

We quickly became inseparable, almost literally joined at the hip.

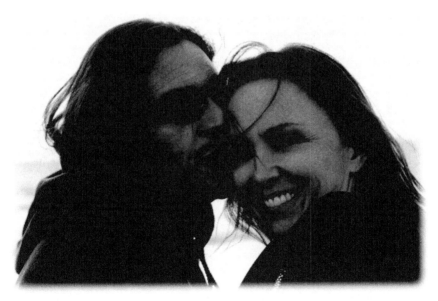

Mario and Liz, Inseparable

35

At this time, I was so ready for a new roommate. Mario was at my house almost every night, which meant we were paying so much in our combined rents, and the girls had no supervision if he was with me. So I came up with the bright idea of moving my roommate out and Mario and his girls in with me.

I know I sound like a crazy person at this point after just two months of knowing him, but in fact, it seemed to solve several problems. If things went well, we could all rent a bigger place, and the girls could get their own rooms. As a girl who needed to have my own room in my teen years (away from my brothers) I really felt for them and thought it should be a priority.

Only recently did Jasmine tell me that was the worst possible time I could have come into their lives. But in the big picture, perhaps it was the *best* time. Our time together would be their one chance to experience a relatively functional family household.

Inheriting Teenage Girls

Although the girls seemed pleased that their dad was focusing on just one woman, they weren't exactly thrilled about this new situation. They had never seen their dad so in love and had always had him in their corner. It would be somewhat terrorizing when the one functional parent who is always there for you suddenly transfers his affection to someone else and doles it on her constantly. His daughters had always come first before other women, but things were about to change... dramatically.

With my experience having stepmothers and stepfathers, I felt I was a good fit for them since I too had a father who played the field, so I could relate. My parents divorced when I was 9 years old, and I threw all kinds of tantrums, especially when my dad remarried a year later.

Still, being thrust into a world of teenagers you didn't raise can seriously test your patience. I tried to make my home comfortable for them; a 2 bedroom, one bath apartment in Venice, 7 blocks from the beach. It worked for a few months but it wasn't easy.

Not long after meeting Mario, he became employed by another general contractor. The more I got to know him, the more I fell for him. Everyone thought we were crazy in love and sickening with our public displays of affection. Trying to dampen that Latin fire is futile. It wasn't just his affection and adoration that drew me to him. It was his huge heart and the way he always showed enthusiasm about other people's victories. It was the way he saw the world, how he felt about religion and spirituality, how he felt about common sense, people and animals. We would

37

watch movies and he could cry at the drop of a dime with no shame whatsoever. I respect that. We were just highly compatible on many levels.

One of the things I loved most was that Mario wasn't into sports, so I never had to lose him to the boys and their games. He preferred just hanging out with me. He enjoyed cleaning, organizing, shopping, all of it. Being a single dad agreed with him and definitely kept him on his toes, as he was a take-charge kind of man.

So when Super Bowl Sunday rolled around, we actually spent that afternoon detailing my car. It hadn't been that clean since I bought it almost 5 years earlier. It was so clean, I remember thinking, "I'm surprised Jasmine hasn't tried to take it out." She always asked if she could drive, and I always said yes so she could get the practice.

What I didn't know was Jasmine *was* in fact borrowing the car frequently after we went to bed. That took serious 'cojones' on her part because I was not *her* mom, and it was not her mother's car. It was mine.

Two nights after the Super Bowl, Mario's then 14-year old daughter, Adelina, woke us up when she was worried because Jasmine wouldn't return her calls or texts. Once we were awake at 3 a.m. only to discover she took my car, we were livid. He called her and told her to get home *immediately!* That scared her so badly that—you guessed it—she slammed it into reverse so fast, that she not only *totaled* my car, she even took out another car in the street and totaled that too. Thank God no one was hurt.

What made me saddest of all was that I had only 5 payments left and 50,000 miles left on my warranty. Luckily, Mario's other car, the Chrysler 300C became mine. He felt responsible for his daughter's actions, but I hated to drive it because the windows were so short, my visibility was compromised. We therefore sold it and put that money down on a Lexus SUV.

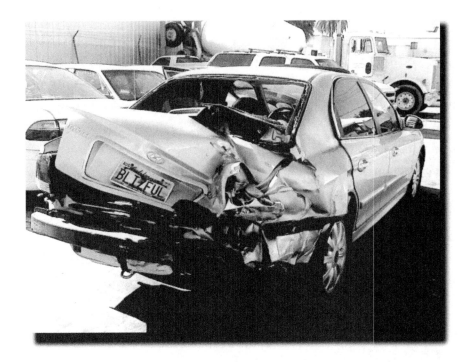

Teenage Joyride - Car Casualty 2010. Not so BLIZFUL

It was a 2004 RX 330 and it was my dream car. Even though I would come out of this fiasco with another 5 years of car payments, I eventually became a *very* happy camper. This new family car would soon come in *quite* handy.

A Not-So-Immaculate Conception

The following month, sometime around mid March, we both attended Costa Acupuncture, our local community acupuncture clinic for Mario to receive treatment for neck pain. While I was in the waiting room, the owner Michael told me that Mario was in a "fertility circle." His other acupuncturist and he had a good chuckle. Hahaha, laugh it up, people!

One of my girlfriends, Audrey Hope, who happened to be in the circle, is a spiritual guidance counselor who also speaks to dead people.

When she had seen a picture of us at Venice Beach during sunset a few months back, she said she "saw a baby around us."

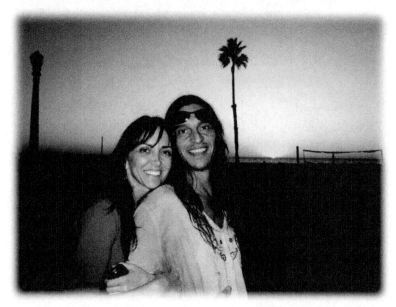

Newly in love, Venice Beach Fall, 2009

40

Mario, having been historically virile, inadvertently contributed to more than one or two pregnant women and had always stepped up to accommodate their choices. But now during acupuncture, he would find himself surrounded by women actively trying to get pregnant, when they had no idea how close they were sitting to 'Mr. Virility.'

Because I have always known

I am a huge wimp when it comes to pain,

I had always been terrified of childbirth.

By the time I was 40, I really wasn't concerned because I assumed my eggs were no longer viable. Yet I was still careful because I wouldn't want to have an abortion. More importantly, I certainly wasn't eager to have a baby from a man who was not 'on board.'

For years I had been on the pill, but at age 36 I finally stopped. My body was rejecting it. I had always used condoms and once in steady monogamous relationships after 36, the pull-out method always worked for me. Mario felt so certain he would not impregnate my 44-year-old body, he started his new hobby of *not* trying to be careful.

His other favorite hobby is eating sweets, so being around him all the time weakened my defenses, which caused my belly to grow. I kept telling him I looked like I was pregnant. He loved to joke, "*I'll* tell you when you're pregnant!"

My period had always come like clockwork, but ... eerily, about two weeks after that fertility circle, I was *late*. When Mario came home with pregnancy tests, I got a little nervous. I had only taken a few in my life, as I had never made the intentional effort to *try* to get pregnant, so naturally the tests always came up negative.

On April 4 I took a test first thing in the morning so I could get the most accurate response. I set it on the sink while I sat on the toilet. We were chatting about the possibilities. A couple of minutes later Mario looks at it and says to me, "You're pregnant." I was certain he was joking. I didn't believe him. He handed it to me, and I didn't see a straight line or a plus sign. I saw the word "Pregnant."

Seeing the word leaves no room for confusion—does the plus mean good? Does the dash mean bad? Good? What? Seeing the actual word really struck me. As Mario recalls, the first words out of my mouth were, "I'm getting an epidural!"

"That's the first thing you think of?" Mario asked in bewilderment. "HELL YES! I think of the PAIN I've been terrified of my entire life because I don't handle pain well," I shrieked.

Every one of my friends who has experienced childbirth has described in great detail the horrors of the pain. Every movie and television show I've seen that dramatized births did a very good job of depicting how painful and terrifying it is, and that we should be in a hospital—just in case something goes wrong. Even if the laboring women had started out wanting to go natural, they are often shown begging for the epidurals, sometimes when it's too late. I always knew if *I* were at the hospital, I saw myself asking for it *immediately*.

I had even started writing a book when I was 35 called *Advice for My Unborn Child*. I thought I had better start compiling life lessons so that if I ever lost my life in the delivery, my child would have a long accumulated list of motherly wisdom to guide it through its life.

Here we were, 44 and 46; together we were 90 years old. We didn't tell anyone for several days. We would lie in bed in shock and talk. It was sort of a 'baby daze.' It's actually a great time in life, wondering what it will be like to meet another human who will be a combination of you and your lover.

We made an appointment with his family doctor in the Palisades and wanted to get the blood test to confirm the facts before we told a soul.

I had already put on about 8 pounds since I met Mario. It's much easier to avoid sweets if you don't keep them in the house. Mario had to have pastries, cookies and cakes around at all times. Much like a hummingbird that survives on sugar water, he has such high energy, he burns through food quickly — but that didn't help *my* girlish figure.

I sometimes wonder if Annie is right — that you can get pregnant more easily if you have extra weight on you. Perhaps women who are particularly thin (like so many in Los Angeles) have trouble conceiving, and then may be forced to opt for the in-vitro fertilization procedures.

This is when things became real.

Here I was, 44 and pregnant. I had no money, no ring on my finger, no health insurance, and no parents around to help. Not that I require a ring on my finger, but we really were still very fresh in our relationship, only having known each other for about 7 months, only having lived together for 5 of those months.

I had never been pregnant, but I also knew that I wasn't emotionally capable of having an abortion. I always knew that if I got pregnant after 40 it would be *fate*, that I was surely meant to have it, that my time had come. After all, I believe we choose our

43

parents, so how could I turn down a soul who had requested me to be its host?

I ran to tell Annie first. She was so excited. She loves babies and she loves *love*. She had raised her two beautiful daughters, Asia and Devin. I often blame the two of them for my pregnancy. When Mario and I were first dating, they were constantly asking us when we were going to have a baby. It was as if we were a celebrity couple that was being prodded to procreate—almost as though they ordered a baby from the universe.

But on this day, I was still not thrilled. I was in a near panic. Annie is so comforting, like a surrogate mommy that any motherless daughter would want to have. She assured me, "Don't worry, Lizzy. Babies, bring good luck!" She followed that with, "Oh my goodness, we're going to have a *baby!*"

At the time I didn't *quite* share her level of enthusiasm. I don't have anything against a woman's decision to abort a baby, and I really didn't feel prepared or equipped on any level for any of this. Still, there wasn't a choice in the matter. I was pregnant for the first time *ever* at 44. It was clearly a matter of fate.

Later, Mario would proudly tell me and other people how he got me pregnant "on purpose." Really, he figured if I got pregnant, he would deal with it. His previous girlfriend was younger than me and she never got pregnant, so why would I? But as it turns out, this baby and I clearly defy the odds, and this wouldn't be the last time.

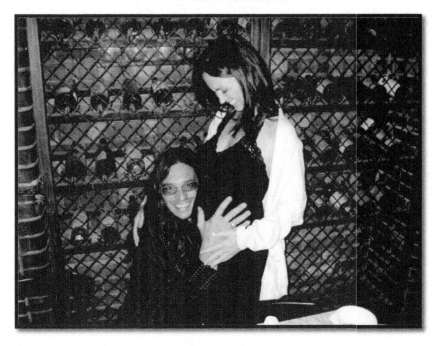

Mario and Liz, Pregnancy Bliss

When it comes to conceiving, there are many great resources you can try, besides acupuncture, besides In-vitro, endless books and websites are at your fingertips.

If you are super slim, maybe put on a *few* extra pounds first. Seek out other sources that bring you joy, try not to stress, trust in fate and let nature take its course.

Above all else, enjoy your relationship while you have the luxury of your freedom and enjoy it while you don't have the added stress of children. Or trust me on this one; there will come a day when you will really wish you had.

If your current challenge is trying to conceive, I have heard amazing success stories resulting from the information in the book *Making Babies — A Proven 3-Month Program for Maximum Fertility* by Sami S. David, MD and Jill Blakeway, LAc. Because my pregnancy came out of left field, I have no personal experience with this book. It came highly recommended by my awesome life coach in Pacific Palisades, Heather Hayward, who we can all thank for urging me to write this book. For those of you *trying* to conceive, Heather enthusiastically recommends *Making Babies* due to its startling success rate.

I feel very good about sharing this resource, mostly because it offers the frame of reference of both Eastern and Western medicine. Our current pediatrician, for instance, is an MD as well as a licensed acupuncturist. She has never needed to use acupuncture needles on our child, but knowing she operates from this foundation of comprehensive knowledge gives me great comfort, because I know she isn't as quick to write prescriptions for antibiotics. In general, I feel doctors who are trained on both sides of the fence are the most knowledgeable and *perhaps* more trustworthy.

The BIG Announcement

Once we got the results of the blood test from the doctor, we knew it was official. The first thing we wanted to do was inform the family.

Mario's mother was visiting us from Colombia, and he wanted to make the announcement at dinner so they would all hear it together—his daughters, his mother, and his brother Sergio. They were waiting on pins and needles for our so-called "big announcement" but to my surprise, none of them had ever even guessed or dreamed it would be *this*. They were all sitting around the table while I was still cooking. Suddenly, Mario shocked the entire family with the announcement. "We're going to have a baby."

Sergio was speechless. Jasmine said, "That's it? That's the announcement? Ok, can I go out now?" Adelina had nothing to say, but just after dinner asked, "I don't mean to be rude, but ..." Yes? "Can we afford a baby?" The actual answer to that was, "No, and we can't afford teenagers either, so it might be time to pack it up." I'm joking, but honestly, I do believe the universe always provides. Why it usually provides *at the 11th hour* is always a mystery to me.

As we were cleaning up after dinner, Mario's then 80-year-old mother asked us if we were serious. She thought the whole thing was a joke. It did seem ridiculous, his being 46 and my being 44—starting a family so late in our lives. But we certainly weren't laughing. One thing was for sure. Our family was about to grow by one.

I began telling my friends and family. All the years leading up to this, whenever I called anyone with big news, they had always asked, "You're getting married? You're pregnant?" No, no, it was always a story about either a move or a new job or career. So this time, at my age, pregnancy or marriage was their *last* guess and my news therefore turned out to be more shocking than anything else.

Each friend met the news with a slightly different reaction. Most were very excited, some were concerned because I hadn't been with Mario that long and they hadn't known him long enough to form an opinion of him as a reliable man or even as a father. What helped his case was the fact he took on sole custody of his teenage daughters. He had the practice. Even though it was only every other weekend, he still had a consistent presence in their lives up until he decided it was time to file for sole custody.

For the most part, it was rather enjoyable seeing the shock on my friends' faces. I often wondered what it would be like to see one of my girlfriends over 40 telling me she is pregnant. Up until I was 47, I was still the only one.

It Could Happen to YOU

I am jumping forward here to share a quick happy story. In January of 2013, I was in Las Vegas with my good friend Dana. It was on that trip that I was finally able to introduce Dana to my other long-time pal. Sonia, my Vegas buddy who formerly lived in L.A., had quite often joined me in painting the town red over the course of many years.

Sonia and Dana had so much in common. They were both the brightest businesswomen I knew, so generous, fun-loving, life-of-the party girls, very spiritually evolved, and both godmothers. What they had most in common was that they had always wanted to be mothers.

That day in our hotel room, they shared their war stories about wanting babies and failing miserably at trying to get pregnant.

Here they were, 43 years old, both had assumed it was over for them and that their time had passed.

Although it was a sad conversation, I always knew they would connect and really relate to each other, so I was excited they finally met.

I felt so badly for them. I assumed their lack of success at something they had each wanted for so long was probably due in large part to their shares of health problems. But I knew one thing for certain; the world would be missing out on two potentially amazing mothers who were both *clearly* designed for motherhood.

Many events soon transpired in the months that followed. To make a long story short, by the spring of that same year, these two 43-year old girlfriends were able to make their own 'BIG announcements!' Yes, you guessed it. They *both* got pregnant – *naturally*!

By December, at 44 years old, two more women delivered healthy boys in the same week – just in time for Christmas.

Dana and Sonia were, at long last, each blessed with their most cherished gifts. For Dana, baby Jax weighed in at 7 pounds, 14 ounces, and in Sonia's corner, baby Andrew, 6 pounds, 13 ounces.

Perhaps their knowing that it could still happen to someone like me (at 44) planted a seed in their subconscious that it wasn't too late for them, after all. This is another reason I felt compelled to write this book.

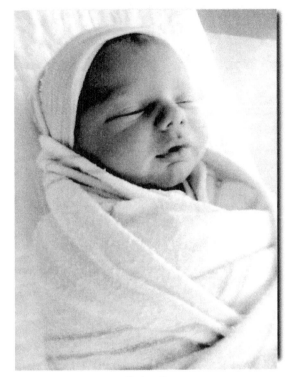

Baby Jax

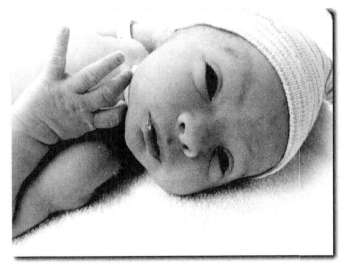

Baby Andrew

Once you see someone do something,

you see that it IS possible,

and if someone else can do it,

maybe you can too!

Think about those statistics they love to pound into our heads. If they say the chances of getting pregnant over the age of 40 are 1-2 percent, and three women in one small group of friends all did it,

maybe we are a lot more capable

than statistics would have us believe.

To give you more hope, since I have spoken to many friends and clients about this book project, I have heard about at least a dozen women over 40 who got pregnant naturally and often unexpectedly. In light of that, I truly believe your baby *will* come if and when it's meant to, but maybe only when you are not panicked about it, or stressing your mates about it either.

However, if you are one who has spent a fortune on in-vitro and is finally pregnant, I feel you are probably the most equipped, possibly the most prepared and perhaps the *most* deserving to be parents.

ACT II

Making Womb

for a New Mom

Preparing the Womb

One of my girlfriends, Malia, had previously worked with me at Goodlife.com in 2009, which was a startup website directory for all things sustainable, spiritual and healthy in Los Angeles. Very excited to learn I was pregnant, Malia wasted no time in turning me on to a natural product that I truly believe affected the outcome of my baby's stellar health. She told me about a product called *Quinton*. It has the same 72 minerals from the sea that are in our blood.

We are all connected by similar makeup, including plants, animals, food and the earth. Malia shared with me that Rene Quinton had done a study of several women who had had four or five miscarriages. He put them all on the minerals and they all proceeded to have healthy pregnancies and, of course, healthy babies. OriginalQuinton.com.

A book that best explains the efficacy of Quinton is called *Brighton Baby* by Dr. Roy Dittmann. A *very* thick book, it's brimming with information, as *"A Revolutionary Organic Approach to Having an Extraordinary Child."*

Because this information is so compelling, I will include this elaborate excerpt from **Brighton Baby--The Complete Guide to Preconception and Conception:**

"The primal communication of our cells is an oceanic rhythm. All sea life pulses with the rhythms of the ocean's tide in sync with the cosmic pulse. When you walk along the sandy beach you can feel this original pulse of life in each wave. Likewise, how our bodies have a mini–ocean of life that reflects this universal reality. All musical

expression has its origins in the ocean's waves and in our mother's aortic pulse that danced through us when we were nestled in her womb. The instinct to rock a baby, the practice of rocking oneself in a rocking chair, or even swinging on the swing reconnects us to this primary rhythmic pulse of life. To humans, returning to the ocean regenerates our primal rhythmic brain. It reawakens our physical, sensual, rhythmic relationship to the earth and the universe. The ocean is the actual planetary womb; a woman's womb is reflexive of this original womb from which all life emerged. That is why people are coming to the correct conclusion that to defile our oceans and beaches is akin to defiling our own mother, because the ocean is the mother of all mothers. Without our oceans, all life would cease to exist. (Balboa Press, Dittmann p. 76)

In the womb, your internal ocean quite literally will direct your future child's brain's development. (Dittmann, p. 77)

The famous French scientist (1866 to 1925) Rene Quinton, proved to the world in 1897 that seawater extracted from certain parts of the ocean may just answer the question about what is evolving life on our planet today. René Quinton saw these hurricane–like swirls of life in the oceans. He theorized that this unique part of the ocean was like the amniotic fluid of the sea. His theory was that all life either began or evolved in this fluid.

To demonstrate this theory, he conducted an experiment in front of hundreds of medical doctors, where he drained the blood out of a stray dog and replaced it with his isotonic marine plasma. Not only did the dog survive, it thrived. This experiment is known to have been independently repeated more than five times throughout the 20th century, each time confirming the same results: marine plasma is a precursor to red and white blood cells.

Before life began, the ocean was filled with a "soup" of elements from the Periodic Table. As time progressed, these elements mixed with organic (nonliving) molecules from the undersea vents. This enriched "soup" was then organized and enlivened by an energy source (e.g. sunlight, cosmic rays, a meteor, lightning, etc.), which gave rise to life.

At some point, a radical transformation took place where higher, more sophisticated life forms evolved on our planet. Quinton asserted that if this was true, then our blood must be a kind of internal ocean. (Dittmann, p.78)

Indeed, Quinton demonstrated that this special seawater could be used effectively as a blood plasma replacement. He called his special seawater Plasma de Quinton ("Quinton's plasma"), now simply referred to as Original Quinton. Marine plasma is the viscous fluid produced by zooplankton as they eat phytoplankton produced inside these vortex plankton blooms. Rene Quinton never fully knew why the fluid he extracted from these zones was so special. He just observed species of marine life traveling from thousands of miles away to reproduce and feed in this special seawater. He knew that these life forms depended on the nutrition somehow uniquely contained in the center of this bloom.

Quinton's profound discovery forever transformed emergency medicine, pediatrics, and perinatal medicine around the world. In the early 1900s, Original Quinton's safety and efficacy was documented in hundreds of thousands of cases. In fact, 69 free clinics known as "Marine Dispensaries" were established throughout Europe and Northern Africa where Plasma de Quinton was administered for dozens of life threatening health conditions.

The efficacy of Original Quinton is due to its abundant, biologically accurate information. Dissolved and recorded within the sea, there is a record of everything that has ever lived on our planet. There are genes from all living species that are living now and that have ever lived on our planet in seawater. In Original Quinton you are getting a complete record of living history; it is teaching your cells adaptive biochemistry. (Dittmann, p.79)

To demonstrate the elegant simplicity of marine plasma, Rene Quinton built his legacy taking on impossible reproductive challenges. Under the direction of Dr. Jean Jarricot, women would come to the clinic with a history of multiple failed pregnancies or a history of severe birth defects, including under-developed infants that died in early childhood. Dr. Jarricot would give Marine Plasma to these women *before and during their next pregnancy. In almost every documented case, the next child would be born healthy. He carefully documented hundreds of these pregnancy cases, following the children sometimes into early adulthood.*

Why is it so effective?

Original Quinton seems to correct the way in which our genes are being expressed at a fundamental level. After all, everything you see in nature – including the complex intelligence stored in your genes – is nothing more than an intelligently organized bundle of elements from the Periodic Table. It is increasingly recognized that genetic transcription depends heavily on the presence of trace elements. Marine Plasma contains all of the naturally occurring elements on the Periodic Table – giving your future baby control over its own perfect evolution within the womb. How Marina Plasma informs our genes is not something that science fully understands. And yet, the clinical case studies tell us all we need to know – that Quinton's Marine Plasma is communicating something powerful to our genes. It seems to be making corrections in our genetic expression – corrections that may shift your future child's biological destiny. (Dittmann, p.81)

Our cells understand original Quinton, because they learned its "language" when the first cellular blueprint was set. The same cannot be said for many of the processed foods, drugs, and in organic dietary supplements that we consume today on a regular basis that contain structurally damaged and even synthetic ingredients. Like a key that no longer fits the lock, whatever our receptor sites fail to recognize, our immune system rejects, thereby triggering an inflammatory response – a phenomenon that may contribute to chronic degenerative illnesses and infertility.

Even with all factors considered, life is very simple. Even though there is endless complexities and interactions between all of the minerals, gases, vitamins, fats, amino acids, sugars, and microbes in our bodies, our bodies are quite elegant and simple. When we saturate our bodies with the fluids and nutrients ourselves were built around, we return to health." (Dittmann p.82)

I took *Quinton* without fail, every day of my pregnancy. When we went to get the 4-D ultrasound, the doctor told us that our baby was "developing beautifully and had a very thick neck" which meant it was *not* at risk for Downs Syndrome (DS). Therefore, the doctor said he *"would not dream* of recommending amniocentesis." I don't believe I would have elected to do that, but I am *very* happy I wasn't faced with that decision. He told me they only recommend it if you have a 1 in 100 chance of having a DS baby, and he told me my chances were roughly 1 in 375.

The March of Dimes website says:
At 30, the risk of having a DS baby is 1 in 1,000.
At 35, the risk is 1 in 400.
At 40, the risk is 1 in 100.
At 45, the risk is 1 in 30.

But here at 45, the doctor tells me my chances were 1 in 375? **I personally think that makes the investment in Quinton *worth the risk* for your growing fetus!**

I also suspect *Quinton* may have affected the outcome in that I had no complications whatsoever. I didn't even have stretch marks, although I have been told stretch marks are most likely hereditary. However, I do believe it may have prevented me from having any morning sickness or cravings. I read that cravings during pregnancy are caused by a sodium deficiency, which is why so many women crave pickles. Since there is plenty of sodium in the sea minerals I took daily, that might explain the absence of cravings.

I also took *Quinton* every day after my pregnancy until I stopped nursing.

No-Stress Express

Indeed I was blessed to have a relatively stress-free pregnancy. This was largely due in part to the fact that Mario landed a substantial construction project, which carried us through the first year of our child's life. It was just like Annie predicted; "Babies bring good luck!"

Within just a day or two of pregnancy confirmation and sheer panic over our lack of money or insurance, Mario got a call from an ex girlfriend who had married a director and needed to remodel their new house in Santa Monica Canyon. Right away, there it was . . . the universe *always* provides!

I was still massaging and working for the magazine, but it was becoming increasingly more stressful. From all I had read, that was one thing I did not want to be during pregnancy — *stressed*. Mario generously offered to pay for all of our expenses so I could just relax and provide our new addition with the most stable and serene womb possible.

I quit my job and that summer we took a much-needed vacation, which was my first proper vacation in nearly ten years. We decided to go to Jamaica.

By the time we left for vacation, I was 5 months pregnant. I was gaining weight rather quickly and my body was expanding. I had never gained weight before, outside of 5-10 pounds. My body was the biggest it had ever been. I had a very difficult time walking around. My sacrum also seemed to be growing to accommodate my ever-expanding ass, that helped support my growing belly.

The sciatica that ensued was probably the most painful part of my pregnancy—if you don't count the labor. I celebrated my 45th birthday in Jamaica, and each step I took was nearly excruciating. Middle age was wreaking havoc on my body and my aches and pains made me second-guess my decision to move forward with this plan.

We had a very relaxing trip, if you don't count the news that our friend watching the house called us about the teenagers, parties and cops. *Again?* Can't we leave town even once with no incident? I decided not to focus on that. I simply focused on happy thoughts, reggae music, friendly people, and watching good comedies.

After having seen shows like *Teen Mom* and *I Didn't Know I was Pregnant* and hearing about all the problems so many women have prenatally, during delivery and postpartum, I felt as safe as a woman could be. I was getting excellent care and I was in good hands at home with my loving man. Honestly, aside from boredom and exhaustion, the most agonizing part of the pregnancy was choosing a name for our baby to come.

No Shame in a Name

Choosing the name is part of the fun, but what's not fun is sharing the news with any family or friends before it's even born. You think you're going to get them prepared for the idea, but they all chime in with their whines and pleas for other options. You become so weary from the dirty looks and grimaces, you begin doubting your own decisions. Even after you've both finally agreed on something you like, you still don't like when your final choice is met with furrowed brows. You might consider not telling a soul until after the baby is born.

We had initially chosen a very unconventional name, but we both loved the sound of it. You've heard of the name *Seven*, mentioned on *Seinfeld*. And we loved the name *Devin* (Annie's youngest daughter) and we loved the number 11. We decided to name our child *Eleven* regardless of its gender. It had such an excellent flow with Mario's last name, *Ayala*. *Eleven Ayala*. It has a nice ring and a poetic flow to it, right?

Half of our friends loved it. The other half, mostly family, thought we were totally crazy and begged, "Can't you please give the baby a name that isn't so nutty, so confusing for people, and is a *name* and *not a number*!?"

Mario is all about doing what he wants and not worrying about what "other people think." I'm a little more concerned with what people think, because those people are not just affecting how I feel, but will certainly affect how my child will feel. When there is this much adversity from people before it's even written in stone, imagine what our kid might go through *with that name* for *life*. As children, we all endure enough teasing as it is.

Deciding on a name is one thing. Agreeing with your partner is another story. By the time you are in your mid 40's, at least one of you has associated negative connotations with almost every name out there. For many years, I had decided if I had ever had a daughter, her name would be *Ruby Juliet* and I would call her *Ruby Jewels*.

We were thrilled to learn we were indeed having a girl. Mario had always wanted a daughter named *Mia* or *Maya*. He was not particularly interested in *Ruby* and I wasn't especially crazy about *Mia* or *Maya*. Naturally, we each wanted to be excited about the name. Today, our next-door neighbor's daughter is *Maya* and our daughter's two best friends at school are both named *Mia*. Whew! Dodged a bullet there.

The second choice we both agreed on was *Summer*. We still loved the name *Eleven*, so it was going to be *Summer Eleven Ayala*. Then we kept hearing, "Oh, thank heaven for Summer Eleven." These haters annoyed me but I thought it was cool that her initials would be SEA. We lived right near the beach so it seemed fitting.

Not long after conceiving, we relocated to a killer spot in the Marina Peninsula—between the Venice Canal and the Santa Monica Bay—a gem of a find if you can land an affordable space. We got lucky because good places get snatched up so quickly in this town. We struck gold with a 3-bedroom, 2-bath apartment with a fireplace, a dishwasher, a washer and dryer and a huge deck with a view of the beach—just steps away. Mario's daughters finally had their own rooms and now we would have a beach baby! As Charlie Sheen would say, "*WINNING!*"

I digress… Back to choosing the name…

Isabella was our next choice. Not long after that agreement, I learned it was the number one name choice for baby girls. This was probably due to the success of the film *Twilight* and its lead character, Bella. The *last* thing I wanted was another common or trendy name that isn't original at all. I wanted something unique, sort of exotic and rolled off the tongue nicely. After the *Eleven* fiasco, I didn't want anything too crazy or difficult to spell or remember. So there we were, back to the drawing board — once again!

About midway through my pregnancy, I got a call from my friend Audrey — the one who talks to dead people. She told me she received a message that my baby was my mother — coming back to be my *daughter*.

Soon after receiving that call, I took a trip to visit my best buddy, Elizabeth, who lived in Palm Desert. That week I was having relationship struggles. In the past, I would always run away to my mom in those instances. Without her, Elizabeth was my only friend who filled that need. I first met her in court reporting school in 1991 and we've been like soul sisters ever since.

She lived in a great house at the time with a heated pool, so I enjoyed that like nothing else. I was taking the weight off my overly inflated body, while reading a good book in the warm desert sun. It was in that pool that the name finally came to me.

As I was reading, I came across the word 'daisy,' which reminded me it was a name I had always loved. It was that day that I developed the name *Deja Francesca*. Deja is French, like my late mother, and also means "already" as in 'déjà vu' (already seen), which could have multiple meanings - seeing myself as a child again, seeing my mother in her or being her mother again, etc. I have been told that we continually attract the same 'soul groups' into our lives throughout multiple lifetimes again and again, so who knows? Even more fitting, it combined Annie's daughters' names *Devin* and *Asia*, as a tribute to both of them.

I couldn't wait to tell Mario. He thought my name choice was "okay." He didn't really care for *Francesca*. He was still attached to *Isabella*. He finally agreed to *Deja*, and we both agreed on *Isabella* as her middle name. Her initials would be DIA, Spanish for "day."

Since choosing the name I have heard nothing but positive comments about how pretty that name is. Finally! *That's* what I most wanted for her. Everyone who meets her older sisters always mention how lovely their names are and I really wanted the same thing for Deja.

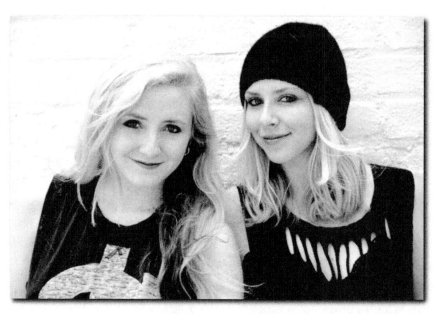

Devin and Asia Moses, Rapper and Singer, Songwriters

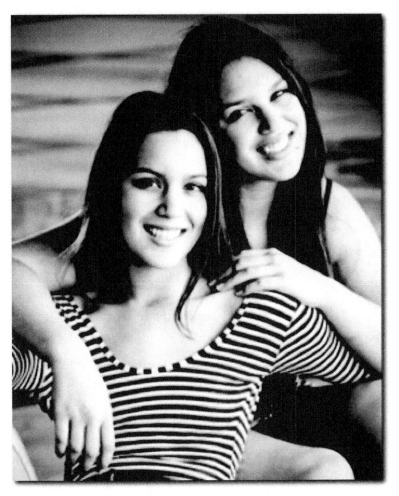

Sisters Jasmine and Adelina Ayala, 2010

On Earth as it is in Heaven

From the very beginning of my pregnancy, I totally cleaned up my act. I stopped all drinking alcohol and smoking pot. I was already a lightweight and barely smoked or drank, but I basically became as pure as the driven snow. I was practically the Virgin Mary. Okay, maybe not a virgin. But my *drinks* were! As I've mentioned, my pregnancy went great. I did not have a single complication and I think I only threw up once or twice, and that wasn't even from morning sickness.

One day I went to my favorite sushi restaurant in Santa Monica for some pot stickers and a Rainbow Roll. Many people think pregnant women shouldn't have raw fish, but I'm not sure if I buy into that warning. I know plenty of moms who did eat it, and now their kids love sushi. What do the pregnant mothers eat in Japan? And don't people in Japan live the longest?

That day at the sushi restaurant, I was really hungry and was saving the best pieces for last. Clearly I had too much on my plate but I finally ate those last delectable bites. As they went down, I knew it was a mistake. I was in trouble. The bathroom was all the way around the restaurant and I wouldn't make it there quickly. I tried to fight it, but I lost the battle. My entire meal was quickly laid out on the sushi bar and the floor beneath me. I was so relieved no one else was sitting at the bar during this late afternoon lunch. There were two cuddling lesbians in the booth right behind me who looked at me very concerned and asked if I was okay.

I don't think my pregnancy was that obvious at the time, so they were probably wondering if it was the food that made me spew. I quickly explained that I was just pregnant and ate too much. I left $10 for the clean up efforts and immediately made my walk of shame directly out the front door. I have since returned to the 'scene of the grime' many times, and luckily no one recognizes me.

Pregnancy leaves you with an endless list of **don'ts** and **can'ts**. When in Jamaica, I really enjoyed the climate and the water, but there was very little I was allowed to do. They wouldn't let me swim with dolphins because they said the dolphins would surround me, as to protect my growing fetus and ignore the rest of the tourists. They wouldn't let me go zip lining, or on a ride through the jungle or much of anything really. I couldn't even ride the slide off the boat. They just kept saying, "That's a precious gift from God, you know, Mon."

As much as I *loved* my hobby of improvisation classes at the Westside Comedy Theater in Santa Monica, I wasn't even able to complete Improv III. It is very physically demanding. I realized at about this stage it was far too strenuous for me. Thinking on your feet with a growing belly makes you even hotter than the heat generated merely from your own self-induced pressure.

One day while I was very bored and stressed during my pregnancy, I had a long talk with my neighbor who was a yogi, a DJ and a beautiful young mother of a toddler. Like so many in California, she was a card-carrying member of medicinal marijuana.

She confessed to me that she vaporized while she was pregnant. I thought that was brave and kind of her to share this information with me. At that time, all I could notice was how mellow her baby was. I had always been amazed that I never heard her daughter really cry or scream, like you would expect from most babies, especially toddlers.

I then decided to do some research. In fact, they ran studies in Jamaica about women who smoked while pregnant. The test concluded that women who smoked had healthier babies than the mothers who did *not* smoke.

When she was alive, my mother revealed to me that she drank and smoked cigarettes through all three of her pregnancies. At the time I don't think anyone knew how dangerous that was. Somehow my siblings and I were all born in perfect health. Not that I am condoning any of *that*, but it did make me think.

As a product of the 60's, born and bred in Sonoma County, I have been exposed to some of the country's best wine and weed for all of my adult life. Several of my classmates grow plants on their properties and some own vineyards and wineries. As a bit of a 'tree hugger,' I have a strong belief in the natural healing powers available to us from Mother Earth. I believe in the resveratrol and other healing properties from our grapes—as I believe in the dozens of health benefits many have gained from the *proper* use of our herbs.

I kept hearing that what helps the mother helps the baby. If you are stressed, that is probably the worst thing for them. On the other hand, when you are happy and relaxed, that is *optimal* for the baby. I have heard from multiple mothers that many OBGYNs will tell you *in confidence* that one glass of wine is fine while pregnant.

As I am a believer in moderation, I wondered if a tiny bit of vaporized marijuana could relax me as much as a glass of wine would. Could it even be healthier than wine? I also wondered if we are told not to do things like have alcohol because so many people out there don't know when to stop. One drink might lead to the next and the next. For some, it can be like giving sugar to kids, creating a desire for more and more. But for a reasonable mother who has the wherewithal to stop at one glass of wine, or one puff in times of stress, could that be okay? *Who* would be the authority to declare if minimal vaporizing or having a bite of a medicinal brownie might be an equally safe choice? I scoured the web for whatever I could find.

Most of the information I could find on Marijuana has to do with low sperm count or difficulty with conception. I found an article in The March of Dimes website that using marijuana while pregnant may cause premature birth, low birth weight or neonatal abstinence syndrome (where the baby goes through drug withdrawal after birth).

The news recently reported that Americans are now smoking more marijuana than they are drinking alcohol. If that is the case, it makes you wonder what mothers-to-be might be doing behind closed doors.

Because of its proliferating popularity, CNN recently aired the special *WEED* where Dr. Sanjay Gupta documented the good and bad effects of cannabis. For some it appears to be very helpful for multiple ailments and for others it can cause highly undesirable effects. I am told a lot depends on the strain used, but most depends on the individual, as we are all unique. Dr. Gupta reported the important fact that a person's prefrontal cortex is not fully developed until the age of 25. This would be a helpful fact to share with teenagers!

It's no secret that the U.S. is a very fear-based country and people who are against it are particularly passionate about it. Those not against it seem afraid to press such a hot button with regard to pregnancy. As long as it is not legal in every state, they will never run the type of studies here that they did in Jamaica. If you are avidly against cannabis because you believe it is a dangerous drug, this is a moot point.

Still, at the critical time of birth, hospitals pump all sorts of synthetic drugs into women when they are in labor, and *that's* okay? They will tell you when you are pregnant that Tylenol is about the only thing you can take *safely*. Still, Tylenol is man-made, doesn't grow in the ground and taking too much can cause liver damage.

With so many variables and life circumstances, every mother-to-be has to decide for herself what she will or won't do and devise her plan on how she will calm herself while carrying her baby. I do believe a lot more is going on than what is being openly discussed.

In the meantime, I found some alternatives you may like to try. I have read that banana tea can be very calming. If you cut off the top and bottom of the banana and steep it in boiling water for 3 minutes and run the hot water through a sieve, you can get three or four times more magnesium from drinking it than from eating it. One of my favorite relaxation aids is Calms Forte, a mild sleep aid which works for me like a homeopathic Xanax. Another remedy I love is Dr. Schulze's Nerve Tonic, which you can order online.

Obviously, if you can remove stressors from your life while pregnant and can remain calm and relaxed with natural forms of healing, you are in the zone. Just remember that

breathing deeply will always be

your best course of action

to relax in any stressful time.

For those 9 to 10 months, your ideal scenario is resorting to meditation and yoga, remaining completely clean and sober during your entire pregnancy, and visualizing a healthy happy baby.

70

I have found that the more I veer towards nature, the more I feel in sync, in general. In the YouTube documentary *Grounded* by Kroschel Films, modern man shares the ancient wisdom that we can heal ourselves simply by walking barefoot or regularly connecting directly to the earth. In an experiment in one small town in Alaska, people healed from all sorts of ailments like chronic pain, stress, snoring, and inflammation *just* by becoming grounded. One woman in the film mentioned having been very sick for the first few months of her pregnancy before she started living 'grounded.' Had I known this at the time of my pregnancy, I might have had more energy! I would have spent more time on the beach, burying myself in the sand or walking barefoot on the grass.

This year I felt very lethargic with many aches and pains. Lately, I have spent more time walking barefoot on the grass and noticing a marked improvement in how I feel — particularly on the days I do that.

I have recently become privy to a book that seems to have had a miraculous effect on many people, *Healing Back Pain* by John E. Sarno, MD. Evidently, after identifying stress and other psychological factors in back pain, he demonstrates how many of his patients have gone on to *heal themselves* without exercise or other forms of physical therapy. I love this concept.

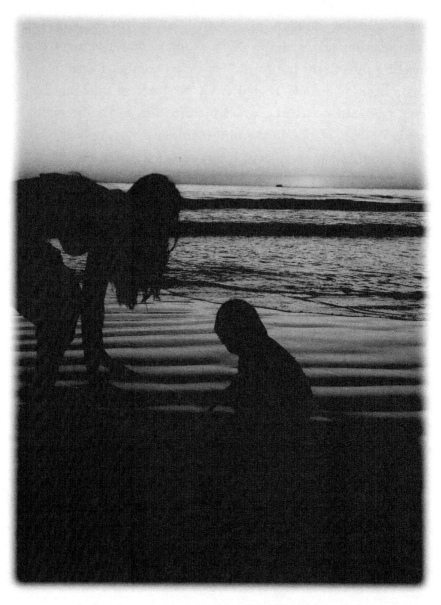

Me with future Deja – Santa Monica Beach, 2012

From High Risk to Warm Water

When the time had come to seek out a doctor to deliver the baby, I asked around. A friend of mine had recommended an OBGYN at Saint John's Hospital in Santa Monica. I had hoped to deliver my daughter in my favorite town, so this seemed ideal. The fact that her name was Dr. Bliss made me wonder if we were being divinely directed. She was a very pleasant woman with lovely energy.

We were faithful about attending our appointments. We were told because of my age that I was "high risk." These statistical labels may hold some validity to them, but I couldn't go there.

I refused to buy into the

label of being called "high risk."

I didn't feel *that* old and I had always taken good care of myself. I had always paid attention to eating as healthy as I could and I made sure to exercise regularly, whether at the gym or just walking every morning outdoors. People have always told me I looked young (as they did my mother) so I probably just lucked out with youthful genes.

Honestly, I usually attributed my youthful appearance to the fact that I had not been married with children. I was able to sleep in almost daily, soaking up my beauty rest, year after year. It's clear to me now that nothing will age you faster than the stress, the drudgery and sleeplessness that come with having *children*.

I don't know how many prenatal appointments we had before realizing they were becoming predictable. With each appointment, there was a good hour-long wait, which grew increasingly uncomfortable as my body grew. The stress of the about-to-expire parking meter only added to my irritability. What didn't help matters was the constant stream of pregnant women waddling in and out of the office who seemed to have shorter waits than we did.

Once we finally got in to see the doctor, our visit would conclude with her comment, "Okay, everything looks great!" The invoice that soon followed was for nearly $400. What the cost of those very short visits entailed, we couldn't comprehend or justify.

One weekend, Mario treated me to a luxurious spa get-away at Two Bunch Palms out in the desert. They had so many great treatments there like mud baths — which of course, I was prohibited from because of my pregnancy. Yet another *don't*.

I did, however, thoroughly enjoy the natural hot spring pools. Heaven! In those two days we enjoyed 11 treatments, and my most memorable was the *Watsu* (water massage). It's basically a Thai Massage in the water where they stretch you and manipulate your body in a mineral pool.

When you are pregnant, little can feel more wonderful. I think it's because the water feels like you are joining your baby's experience in a womb outside the womb. Weightlessness is blissful during pregnancy. The woman who performed the treatment assured me my "baby was *loving* it!"

I mentioned I had considered having a water birth and she told me I should really look into it, that it's definitely the best thing for the baby and continued with her reasons. That got me thinking.

When we went back to our room we decided to Google "water birth" and came across the website for the *Sanctuary Birth Center* in Los Angeles, just 10 minutes from our house. They offered a "Meet the Midwives" day, so we considered that.

On our next prenatal visit to our doctor, we mentioned to our doctor that we were *thinking* about a water birth and asked her for her opinion. She clammed up instantly and had nothing to say, no reason to recommend or advise against it—she just said, "I don't know anything about that," and quickly dismissed the subject. Shortly thereafter, we received another $400 invoice.

It didn't take long before we finally got around to 'meet the midwives.' It was very interesting to hear from each midwife about her experience, as well as from the other pregnant couples in attendance. I mentioned that my biggest problem was my serious phobia when it comes to pain.

One of the most seasoned midwives, Racha, told me that in her experience, the ones who can bear pain the least are usually the ones who deliver the fastest. She recalled a past client with a very low pain threshold whose labor didn't last more than five hours. I said, "That's for me! I'm all over that 5-hour labor!"

I also asked about the pain. "Is there no way to get an epidural *and* deliver in the water? Another midwife Katie answered,

"The water acts as sort of an aqua-dural."

Of all the things I learned that day, that was the one comment that made the most sense to me. Each time I have a period with dreadful cramps, the most soothing forms of relief include a heating pad, a hot bath or a hot water bottle.

The midwives further compelled me by explaining that they wait until the baby is *ready* to come. There is no inducing or rushing the baby to meet their agendas or schedules. The midwives have the philosophy that everything happens in due time. Babies *know* when they are ready. I loved the idea of this. It seemed the most humane, the most natural, and as you can surmise by now, I always lean on the side of natural — if and when I have the choice. Who wants to be rushed?

They also told us they would be at our homes with us no matter how long the labor lasted — which could take up to three days — cook and clean for us if necessary, and even comfort us through the process with … *massages*? Sign me *UP*!

Once we decided to proceed with the midwives, it was a dramatically different experience. Our prenatal visits went from about 5-10 minutes with the OBGYN to at least 60-90 minutes with the midwives. We could now lounge on comfortable couches with our feet propped up, rather than trying to remain comfortable and patient in those horrible upright chairs in a typical waiting room. We could sip hot tea while the midwives would ask me questions and answer the many questions I had as well.

Their questions were typically: How are you feeling? What have you been eating? How have you been sleeping? How has Mario been treating you? I can't imagine how we could have talked that long, but they really got to know us and seemed to genuinely care. If they didn't care at all, it was an academy-award winning performance. Either way, it wouldn't have mattered. This was definitely more my 'cup of tea.'

This shift in plans would be the beginning of a very eye-opening education for me, as well as a life-altering journey for our family.

Regular Wisdom

Years ago, I had a colonic by a local hydro-therapist in Santa Monica. I was historically irregular. Something crazy happened during one of my sessions. I was so impacted, that the hose came off the machine and was spraying all over the room (just water, *thankfully!*) After some questioning, she deduced that I had "inherited my father's sluggish colon." "That's just great!" I said. "Most people inherit real estate, boats, stocks, and bonds. All I inherited was my mom's soft skin and my dad's sluggish colon. Lovely!"

I actually learned a *very* helpful tip from that hydro-therapist. As she was inserting the hose in my bum, she instructed me to open my mouth as wide as possible. She explained it relaxes the anus. Wow, was she right! Word to the wise: It also helps during the delivery! But mum's the word (the boys don't need to know this).

What finally changed my regularity happened in 2005. My favorite yoga teacher in Las Vegas told me to try aloe vera pills, which worked miracles—that is, until I became pregnant. When constipation returned, my midwife Aleks suggested I try a handful of Chlorella. I took about ten tablets at a time and it worked *every* time without fail. Thanks to Aleks, my constipation became a thing of the past.

Someone at the *Sanctuary* mentioned a documentary by Ricki Lake, *The Business of Being Born.* We rented it on Netflix and then became that much more certain we made the right choice to have a home birth. The film depicts how propaganda programs us to believe we need a hospital to deliver our babies. What I came to understand was that the hospital business truly *is* a racket. They are, of course, in business to make *money*.

One woman in the film makes a great point when she says that women in our culture spend more time researching which car stereo or camera to buy and don't spend the same amount of time getting educated about their birth choices.

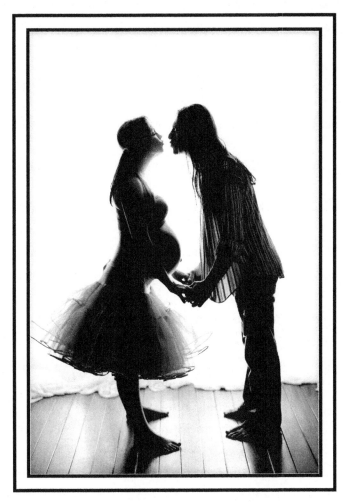

'Lizario' by Lori Dorman Photography

Big Business

Due to the success of *The Business of Being Born* (released in 2008), Ricki Lake and Abby Epstein made four supplemental documentaries—a series called *More Business of Being Born* (released in 2011) also currently available on Netflix.

"The United States has one of the highest maternal mortality rates among all industrialized countries. Today, midwives attend 70% of births in Europe and Japan. In the United States they attend less than 8%."

          -*The Business of Being Born* (BOBB)

Since the early 1900s, the number of midwives attending births went down dramatically. Fortunately, as we become a more conscious society, this number is back on the rise. Midwives have been attending and assisting births since ancient times, until hospitals became industrialized.

Midwives are trained in everything medically to do with the birth outside of surgery. They are fully informed about the mothers who may well be high risk and are fully aware of possible complications. They come to the birth very well prepared with emergency tools and equipment and know what to do if there is a need for an emergency transport. They may also perform as a doula as well.

Doulas, on the other hand, are not medical providers and they do not provide exams. They are there more for emotional and physical support and to provide information—not just for the woman in labor, but also for the friends and family. She is more like your emotional cheerleader, she will give you massages, is there with the couple before going to the hospital, and is your advocate who will make sure your desires are being addressed when you are totally out of it. A doula can also make sure the doctor does not bully a woman into a natural birth, a C-section or episiotomy etc.

"Statistically, the presence of doulas has cut labor times in half. They are there to listen. They understand the physiology of birth. And they also understand hospitals and interventions, side effects of medications, and can help guide you to the process. They will help you by discussing your birth plan and what things may or may not occur, and what you might want to do or not do in those instances. They also support the husbands or partners for breaks, snacks, etc."
-More Business of Being Born (MBOBB)

I learned so much from *The Business of Being Born*. I had already had my own undesirable experiences with western medicine's impersonal and corporate strong arm. Many points mentioned in the films make you wonder.

"They've (the hospitals) told women, 'Come to us. We will take care of everybody's birth. It doesn't matter what kind of birth you want. We are open to anything.' And then you get there, and then you realize, 'No, the hospital system is really set up one way, to handle one kind of birth, and you just get put through that system and it's a fight to try to **not** *get put through that system'."*
-Tina Cassidy, Author of Birth.

"In a hospital, the interventions start when they decide that you need Pitocin and an epidural and maybe more Pitocin, and maybe another epidural, and it can cause a snowball effect, which can actually put the baby in distress, which can actually cause the need for a C-section, which probably would not need to happen at all if you were not on the hospital's clock in the first place."

"Hospitals are businesses to be filled and emptied. They don't want women hanging around in the labor room."
-Patricia Burkhardt, N.Y.U. Midwifery Program

"Many people have described birth as a 'rite of passage,' and it is certainly a life-altering experience, and it can be a beautiful, incredible empowering life-altering experience or it can be a devastating, traumatic, scarring (literally and figuratively) experience."
-Elan McAllister, Founder of Choices in Childbirth

It's powerful to hear from educated doctors, psychologists, authors, who explain things from the other side of the fence. It's good to understand what is happening with your baby when you elect to go along with their recommendations for interventions.

"One of the things that we think happens during the whole labor and delivery process is that the oxytocin neurons start squirting out lots of oxytocin in the brain which is the bonding, protective hormones, and the oxytocin travels in the bloodstream down to the uterus, to start triggering the contractions of labor and that's when the switch to the maternal brain circuits—the mommy brain—gets flipped on, and the whole brain cocktail of hormones and neural chemicals has, for millions of years, been developed to keep the mommy absolutely riveted on protection of the helpless infant...

Pitocin is a synthetic version of oxytocin, that you put intravenously in a woman when she is in labor. However, Pitocin doesn't act as natural oxytocin would in the brain... Sometimes modern medical interventions need to be done, but they also inhibit the natural maternal aggression to protect and nourish the baby right after birth that is normal for mammals and human moms."
-Louann Brizendine, Author of Female Brain

Then, there is the question of love. As I mentioned in ACT I, what I had *most* wanted was "a famous love." Now I was about to learn the ultimate lesson in love.

"Until recently, love was a topic for poets, novelists, philosophers. Today it is studied from multiple scientific perspectives. With mammals in general, there is immediately after birth, a short period of time—which will never happen again—and which is critical in mother/baby attachment. Until recently, in order to give birth, a woman, like all mammals, is supposed to release a complex cocktail of love hormones. As soon as a baby is born when mother and baby are together, both of them are under the effect of a sort of morphine of an opiate, natural morphine we know the properties; they create states of dependency, addiction. When mother and baby are close to each other, it is the beginning of an attachment. But today, most women have babies without releasing this flow of hormones... What about the future of humanity?

If most women have babies without releasing this cocktail of love hormones," he questions, *"Can we survive without love?"* ... *"Today we have to rediscover how easy birth can be. When we don't try to make things too complicated, when ideally there is nobody around but an experienced, motherly and silent low-profile midwife."*
-*Michael Odent, MD*

Just as Ricki Lake and Abby Epstein support any woman's choice for her birth plan, I sincerely feel the same. I merely hope women get as informed as possible early on, and don't let themselves get bullied into choices they don't truly want.

In their film, a registered nurse named Marcia Castro shared her labor story. When she was in labor on the 4th of July, she was given Pitocin and instantly went from having manageable contractions to horrific pain. This naturally changed her birth plan, which led to her getting Stadol and eventually an epidural.

She says they make it sound so routine, so matter-of-fact, that you don't even question it yourself. She feels guilty talking about it when she has a healthy child because people will dismiss it and say, "Well, at least he's healthy."

Because her baby was born on a holiday and the hospital was understaffed, they did what they wanted to do ultimately, not because a C-section was necessary but because that's what they chose for her. Six years later she still feels robbed of that experience, which is something she says she will never get back.

"Maternity Care in the United States is in crisis. It's in many ways, a disaster. . . When the baby goes to the birth canal it is squeezed, its lungs are squeezed so much that when it takes the first breath, it fills those lungs. In a C-section the baby is taken out and its lungs are filled with fluid and the air hits all that fluid and there is a significant increase in respiratory distress syndrome in newborn infants where they cannot breathe and they suffocate. Another increased risk from C-section is childhood asthma . . .

*Today in the United States, we **know** that there is serious increase in minimal neurological problems in children and in attention deficit disorders, in autism; all of these things are increasing at the same period of time that we are increasing all of these obstetrical interventions. And we don't know – and maybe next year or next decade, we will discover to our horror, that what happens at birth is very important to the future development of that child."*

-Marsden Wagner, MD

One of my recent massage clients with 9-year old twin boys shared that when she told her sister-in-law (an OBGYN) that she was having twins, she immediately told her, "Okay. You're having a C-section. It's too dangerous otherwise. Trust me."

I thought C-sections were for emergencies. Is this what the medical community is telling all women? If this is what they tell their own families, it makes you wonder.

"In the last 12 years, the Cesarean Sections rate has doubled."

"A growing crisis that is developing is that OBGYNs are choosing C-sections because there are fewer legal problems with them."

"What many doctors won't tell you is that induction can double your chance of having a C-section."

-The Business of Being Born

In *MBOBB* Molly Ringwald had one of the most brave and interesting birth stories. Ringwald was told she was 'high risk' for many legitimate reasons such as being borderline diabetic, having had a late-term miscarriage, a myomectomy, preeclampsia, she was 41 years old, etc. Yet even with all of the odds stacked against her desire to have a natural birth, something in her told her she could carry twins and deliver them naturally... and she did! With the help of Dr. Michael Johnson at UCLA – Ringwald's son, the second baby, was breech and was born feet first. Johnson, however, was trained to do that. Most doctors sadly are *not*.

Dr Stuart Fischbein, who was actually *my* back-up doctor, and who regularly speaks at the *Sanctuary*, goes on to say, "If we don't teach people how to do vaginal births for strange things, the C-section rate will go up."

"With scheduled Cesareans, you are running the risk of prematurity, due dates are often wrong, ultrasounds can be wrong about the size of the baby and when it's due. It is much safer for the baby to wait until the baby's body sends out the signal that initiates labor. That way you can be much more reasonably sure that the labor is not

premature and that the baby's lungs will be fully developed. A number of babies in the NICU because of prematurity, because of cesareans done too soon is much much higher than it should be. It's ridiculous!"
    -Robbie Davis-Floyd, PhD, The Business of Being Born

Another disadvantage to C-sections is that bonding is hampered when the baby goes to a warmer or to the nursery with the dad. Other risks and complications from C-sections are that incisions often get infected and recovery can be very long and painful.

Just last December, one of my massage clients and my two girlfriends Dana and Sonia were all three pregnant with boys and were all due within a week of each other. They all delivered in hospitals, one at UCLA, one at Saint John's in Santa Monica and the other in Las Vegas. Doesn't it seem rather coincidental and suspicious that all three women were told they needed emergency C-sections?

In middle class

and upper middle class sectors,

the C-section rate in Brazil

is now up to 93%.

Typically, the only women who birth naturally in Brazil are the ones with no money. Are we heading in that direction here in America?

Let's say it's your first baby and you are terrified. The doctor knows this and can easily take advantage of your ignorance and fears and help you rack up a hefty price tag at the hospital—just by telling you it's safer for the baby. Why not? They make more money and they can predict what time they will be home for dinner.

I know there is a time and place for everything, but based on my experience with big business, 'big pharma,' and losing my mother to the failures of western medicine, I probably tend to lean on the more skeptical side.

My friend Dana, for instance, whose C-section was at UCLA, was told her baby was 10 pounds and that they probably wouldn't be able to get his shoulder out without breaking it. He actually weighed 7 pounds 14 ounces. That means they were more than two pounds off in their 'educated estimate.'

Had Dana known that, she said she would have definitely tried to push longer. If they can be that far off on their guess when a woman is in *labor*, it makes you wonder how efficient their system really is. Midwives are notoriously much closer in their estimations of baby weight with no gadgets or equipment outside of a tape measure.

As Lake and Epstein mentioned, since *The Business of Being Born* ended in Abby's emergency transfer C-section, it aptly documents that

we are indeed blessed to have access

to both worlds and both options,

to accommodate any scenario.

Another documentary we rented called *Pregnant in America* corroborates much of the information as well as misinformation and myths discussed in *The Business of Being Born.*

Further outside of the box was another documentary called *Orgasmic Birth*. After having read the book, I just couldn't pass up watching the film. One woman actually has an orgasm as she delivers her child. Again, I put my hand up and exclaimed, "Hallelujah! That's for *me!*" Realistically, it sounds great in theory, but in practice—maybe not so much.

A recent massage client who is a personal trainer specializing in prenatal and post natal fitness, Sarah Ann Corkum-Kelly, told me about a friend of her client, Jennifer Block who wrote a great book called *Pushed*.

"A groundbreaking narrative investigation of childbirth in the age of machines, malpractice, and managed care, **Pushed** *presents the complete picture of maternity care in America. From inside the operating room of a hospital with a 44% Cesarean rate to the living room floor of a woman who gives birth with an illegal midwife, Block exposes a system in which few women have an optimal experience. Pushed surveys the public health impact of routine labor inductions, C-sections, and epidurals, but also examines childbirth as a women's rights issue: Do women even have the right to choose a normal birth? Is that right being upheld? A wake-up call for our times, Block's gripping research reveals that while emergency obstetric care is essential, we are overusing medical technology at the expense of maternal and infant health."*
-Amazon.com

Block's website PushedBirth.com also includes a plethora of information including but not limited to the growing rise in C-sections and the rise in the maternal mortality rate.

You're Doing it Wrong

When you become a new mom, or are pregnant for your first time, you naturally assume everything you are doing is wrong. You can't help but compare yourself to everyone else about every issue under the sun. You will also notice the strong urge people have to give you advice or criticism, most often by those who have never even had children! I secretly envision myself throwing bricks at them.

You might be like me and not have much of a mommy gene. I've never looked longingly at the moms in the parks and ached for that lifestyle. In fact, my daughter is now 4 and I still don't really enjoy going to the park. I've personally never been much of a "kid" person. Even as a child, I found myself more interested in the company of adults. I do love kids and they seem to love me. But I have very short spurts of playful energy.

Once you become a parent and are with small children all day, it is so nice to talk to other parents who make you feel human. I still don't understand why we carry so much guilt about that.

For some reason as a mother, you always have in the back of your mind that you are a bad mom, that other mothers are judging you, that you aren't doing it right, etc. This will probably happen no matter how hard you try or how well you do. Eventually, you *may* stop caring what people think.

During my pregnancy, when I was taking prenatal yoga, the teacher was talking about this "special time of connecting to the baby," I felt like I was missing something. I didn't feel a connection to her soul, her heart, her mind, or anything on that level. I was just plain tired.

Fortunately, when I whined about my woes to my midwife Aleks, she said to me, "That's cool. I didn't feel a connection to my baby either. It's no big deal. You'll have plenty of time for that later." Hearing that from a seasoned midwife that was still nursing her two-year-old daughter made me realize I was doing just fine and could *relax*.

I had another epiphany one day at the *Sanctuary*. There was a young, cute mother-to-be in our childbirth prep class who was complaining about how she didn't feel sexy. The boys were in the other room and we were having "girl talk." She explained, "Her boyfriend is totally attracted to her and wanting sex all the time, but I don't feel sexy!" I felt so bad for her. Then I was stunned to learn she was talking about Mario! I assured her, "*I* don't feel sexy either. And by the way, Mario is nuts! He's not normal. I can't get him off me. He's crazy!" I couldn't figure out how she could compare herself to me, or our relationship, for one second.

Mario is a character. Strangers have even approached him asking if he was a shaman or even Johnny Depp. He is definitely an 'outside of the box' wild man, with the energy of a child, and like Tarzan who can climb trees like a monkey. He is a diamond in the rough, who can be uncouth, vulgar and crude. Even though he has no filter, he still has a heart of gold.

Honestly, no one ever knows the full story about what goes on behind closed doors. The grass always seems greener. But this was a major wake up call. As I had always been in the habit of comparing myself to everyone else, on this day I realized that anyone's mere existence or appearance might make us feel like we are "missing" something, without the slightest clue it is happening. The truth is, no one is missing anything. That would have been a good time for us to drill into our new-mommy minds the mantra that preschoolers learn; we get what we get, and we *don't get upset!*

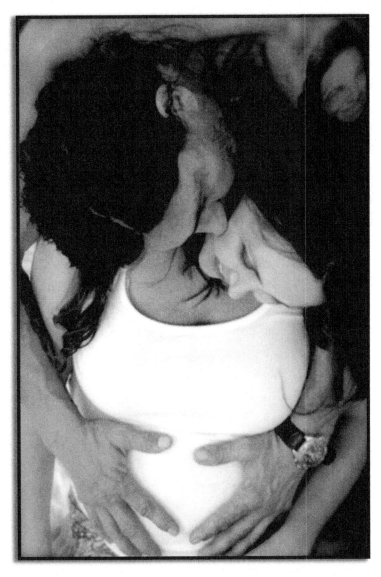

Pregnant and Loved – Photo by Annie Flatley

Yoga Ga Ga

While pregnant, I found exercise just too strenuous. I tried the prenatal yoga classes at Exhale in Venice by Desi Bartlett. She was great. Unfortunately, it was combined with post-natal yoga, meaning new moms attended along *with* their fussy babies. I was about to be subjected to a screaming child, but at this stage of the game I was definitely not ready for that. All it did was *add* to my stress. Instead I took Desi's prenatal yoga video home to practice in peace and quiet.

No matter how hard your man works, at the end of the day, you are exhausted as well. So when he complains about his day or his job, even if you have just been lying around, you can have a bit of fun with him and ask, "Well, what did you do that was so hard?" After he responds you can say, "Really? Well, today I built a liver. Pass me the remote."

The midwives recommended long walks. I took their advice because that was all I could really muster. I was so fortunate at that time to have lived on the beach in an optimal climate. At the very least, I was subjecting my bun in the oven to those awesome negative ions.

In an article featured on WebMD by Denise Mann, *Negative Ions Create Positive Vibes,* Mann explains:

"Negative ions are odorless, tasteless, and invisible molecules that we inhale in abundance in certain environments. Think mountains, waterfalls, and beaches. Once they reach our bloodstream, negative ions are believed to produce biochemical reactions that increase levels of the

mood chemical serotonin, helping to alleviate depression, relieve stress, and boost our daytime energy."

As I grew larger, it became harder to walk up stairs. Mario would often walk underneath me and help push me up *by my big butt!* The one thing I wished I had been more diligent about was working my glutes and leg muscles. As a new mom, you will find yourself forced to bend down much more than usual. Your back will get really worked and sore and can become problematic. It's bad enough when you have a baby in your 40s, your body isn't as strong as it would have been in your 20s or even your 30s.

I am told that for most women over 40, pregnancy is very tiring throughout each phase. In the first trimester all you want to do is sleep. Then as your body grows, you are adjusting to a new size and shape and nothing fits. Even your shoe size will change — maybe even permanently.

Once you are in your third trimester until the time you deliver, discomfort is basically constant. Exercise even for a historically active woman seems a rather dismal prospect.

I personally gained 50 pounds.

Everyone told me it's good to gain weight so I didn't try to fight it. But for someone who was a size 5 for about 30 years, putting on 40% more body weight on a frame of small bones was daunting. Sitting on the couch watching HGTV was far more desirable.

No one needs yoga more than a new mom-to-be, and once your baby comes and that ball and chain has you trapped at home, you are on a new and unpredictable schedule. Having to pack up the baby and the car, drop them at a sitter, get to class, get through the class, pick them up and get back home is an ordeal that will discourage even the most motivated yogi.

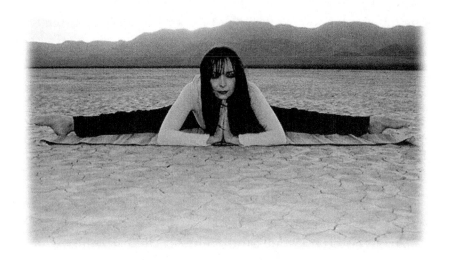

Age 38, Dry Lake Bed Las Vegas 2003

YogaGlo.com was a Godsend. They have a huge library of streaming content with classes as short as 5 minutes and as long as two hours. It's so much easier to access great yoga in the comfort of your own home that you can do while your sweet angel is fast asleep. The best part is, you can pause, rewind, use the bathroom, send a text, or make all kinds of unsavory bodily sounds without considering how you might sound or look. You can filter the search by style, teacher, duration, and even by body part. If you are like me and *need* yoga but can't keep a set schedule or make it to a full-length class, you will *forever* be grateful for YogaGlo.

I am now also very grateful to Power Yoga in Santa Monica. It is a beautiful yoga studio located on 2nd street, which operates on donations. This saved my life during hard times. If you want an easier class that isn't too strenuous, you will enjoy Dan Ward's classes.

My favorite posture for pregnancy takes pressure off of your low back. It's restorative and *so* relaxing. Any inversion fights gravity, sending the blood flowing back up to your organs. If you lie on your back with your legs up against the wall for 15 minutes a day, I'm told it can add years to your life. Consider it a deposit you can make to your 'well-being account.'

Deep breathing is *so* important, physically, mentally and emotionally. Not only is it one of the best tools to help you through your labor—it helps you immensely throughout life. In this fast-paced society, we are all victims of shallow breathing because we are all in constant activity. I have read that oxygen therapy has been successful in curing about every disease known to man, but obviously we don't hear about it because there isn't much profit to be made.

In my practice, I have witnessed what I call a "neck-idemic." We all have our heads down looking at our phones or our laptops and it's wreaking havoc on our spines and neck muscles. You know how they give the nickname "stiffs" to corpses? It's because they *are* stiff. There is no oxygen running through dead bodies, much like the knots we have when we are alive. Therefore, it's my theory that the knots we have in our bodies are basically gasping for air. Feed them every chance you get!

"Life is in the Breath.

He Who Only Half Breathes,

Half Lives."

-Yogi Proverb

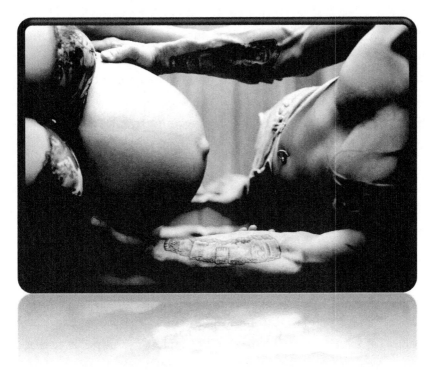

Things to Come
Lori Dorman Photography

A Rainbow a Day

What I enjoyed most was the peace of mind I had, knowing I was putting the absolute best things in my body for myself as well as the baby. The midwives suggested "eating a rainbow every day." That means eat a fruit and/or vegetable of each color of the rainbow to ensure your nutrient and mineral needs are being met.

This part was easy for me because I was already a health nut and knowing it's the best thing for your baby makes it that much more gratifying. Keeping a chart really helped. Anytime after I ate an array of strawberries, blueberries, bananas, cantaloupe and kiwis, I felt a huge sense of pride that I did what I *most* needed to do that day.

My favorite way to meet my rainbow requirement was at our local *Pinkberry*. A dollop of delicious frozen yogurt was topped with every color of fruit I could fit in my cup. It was a delicious treat and the most colorful feast that made me feel so happy — mentally, spiritually and physically — *knowing* I was doing my best job nurturing my yogurt-loving baby to come. The only way it could have been better is if their fruit was organic.

Nesting

Once you realize you have to choose a stroller, a car seat, a crib, bassinet, co sleeper, nursing chair, a baby monitor, etc. *before* the baby comes, it becomes rather overwhelming for a first-time mom.

When it comes to nesting and preparing your home and car for the tiny hurricane that will change everything in its path, there are endless details to consider. Having mom friends nearby who have 'been there/done that,' *really* helps.

First, the baby shower will be instrumental in stockpiling the necessities. I recommend asking a friend who is a fairly recent mother to take you to *Babies R Us* or *Target*. She can help you sort through the goods, letting you know what you *really* need, and what might be a waste of money.

Once you have acquired your new baby needs, you will have storage and organization concerns. But as you are about to pop, you will probably be huge and exhausted. This is when you need to enlist the help of yet another mom friend to help you organize and Feng Shui your closets and cupboards to keep the necessities at arms reach and put away what you won't need until a later date.

As a certified practitioner, I've read dozens of books on the subject and have experienced the energy shift first hand. Good Feng Shui makes a huge difference. Clutter is extremely draining. As a new mom, you are in your home so much of the time, constantly looking around at everything. Each item you see that needs to be moved or stored is just weighing down your energy. You may need muscle to assist you in this process.

What I highly recommend to get you through it is an excellent book by Karen Kingston called *Clear your Clutter with Feng Shui*. It's small and concise, but really packs a punch. In fact, I gifted this book to two girlfriends who desperately needed it. They both reported that it changed their lives dramatically.

Acquiring the Goods

What I recall being most important was the right stroller. It had to be durable but still light enough for me to handle on my own. I needed to open and close it easily enough to get it in and out of the trunk. I also learned that a critical feature is its ability to lie completely flat so the baby's spine can stretch out for optimal growth.

We ultimately chose the iCoo partly because it was affordably under $500, when so many out there are in the $1,000 range—but also because it was built with German engineering. What a great decision that was. Four years later, it is still as sturdy and durable as it was when we first bought it—just a lot less clean. We chose red because when you are crossing busy intersections, you want drivers to *see* you!

There are probably hundreds of different cribs on the market, but in the beginning we didn't even need a crib. Deja slept with us in our bed for the first couple of weeks. You may be cringing at that thought. I was a tad concerned at first, until I learned early on that Deja would not die quietly. Whenever she was the least bit disturbed, she would communicate that swiftly and *loudly*. Some things never change.

After the first two weeks, what worked the best for me was a co-sleeper that sits up high by the edge of your bed so you can nurse or feed the baby and roll it right into its own bed and still give you room to stretch out and cuddle with your honey.

What I loved most about the co-sleeper is that it is narrow enough to wheel through the doorway into another room so you can have some privacy, watch a movie or have some *bow-chicka-*

wow-wow time. We finally got a crib somewhere between 5-8 months. I would estimate that you can keep the baby safely and comfortably in a co-sleeper until it is on solid foods, so you have some time if you want to stretch out your dollars—not blowing your entire wad in the beginning.

Many new moms get into decorating and preparing a baby's room. I would have really enjoyed that if I had the space, the extra cash and the energy. Obviously, it's no secret that a new baby costs a pretty penny. All of the accouterments can create a clutter fiasco. So, in the interest of good feng shui, I think it's always best to keep things as bare and simple as possible.

Once you realize this simple truth, you come to realize how important it is to have a proper baby shower. Not all of us have parents or siblings, grandparents, or cousins who can help with the load. If you are lucky, maybe you have a lot of friends. Obviously, the more people you invite to your shower, the better chances you have of meeting your child's first needs.

I had my baby shower at a trendy Mexican restaurant in the Century City Mall—it seemed ideal since it was in fact, the *Pink Taco*. After all, it would be only two months before this tiny human would emerge from my *own* pink taco. I decided to make it co-ed so it wasn't too girly, and so my male friends could come and everyone could have cocktails if they wanted to drink. It turned out to be a pretty good time. Our celebrity couple name is *Lizario* so Angela had that put on our cake.

I was very blessed to have been gifted many necessities like a nursing chair, a video baby monitor etc. My nursing chair was and still is my favorite piece of furniture. It was a splurge, as I wanted it to be cute, inviting, and as comfortable as my bed is, because I knew nursing was about to become my full-time job. When you nurse exclusively, you are easily spending 8 hours a day at it, so shouldn't you be comfortable?

After trying out all the chairs around town, I found one chair at a high-end baby store that ruined me for all other chairs. Not only was it a rocker and a recliner, it also swiveled. I did my research on it, and called around trying to find it at the best price, and ordered it in pink with white piping. I still love to rock Deja in it and read to her, as it is a source of happiness and comfort for the both of us.

I always find myself buying new moms the Diaper Genie, because although it's not a glamorous gift, it's what every mom needs if they are going to use disposable diapers and they don't want their house to smell like baby poop.

What I discovered most people prefer to buy and bring to the shower is not necessarily what you put on your baby registry, but rather the cutest clothes they can find. The smaller the clothes, the cuter they are (but quite often too small). Even if they go to the store to get something specifically on your registry, they are highly likely to get distracted and compelled to bring you their oh-so-adorable finds.

We almost never spent money on clothes because they kept popping up every time someone would pay a visit and meet our new child.

Clothing Swaps

When Deja was just a few months old, I discovered the most brilliant idea ever; clothing swaps. The first swap I attended was sponsored and organized by Zulily.com.

Another is a regular bi-annual clothing swap hosted by a Yahoo group I belong to called *Venice Moms*. You take a bag of clothes your child has outgrown and then you pick up used clothes from the pile that is your child's current size.

When children are very young, they don't care what they wear, so that's all on you. You dress them in whatever you are not embarrassed to have your child wearing. Newborns outgrow clothes so fast there isn't enough time to wear them out or sometimes even at all, so they are usually in good shape—often brand new.

Once your child is two or three, that's when the selection is rather dismal. The clothes become more stained, faded, tattered and at that point the clothing swaps aren't as useful as they are for the first year or two. I can honestly say that we spent well under $500 on clothing for her entire first two years. Occasionally we bought some new pajamas or clothing sets at Costco, but never needed much more than that. Hand-me-downs from other savvy moms are also *extremely* helpful.

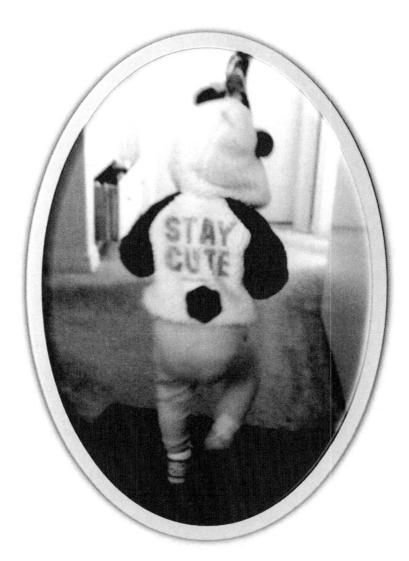

Deja's Diapered Booty

Cloth Diapers

Another big money saver was the use of cloth diapers. I'm told it can cost about $200 a month for disposable diapers. The *Sanctuary* sold colorful soft cloth diaper sets by *GroVia*. We invested about $100 on our supply and a few friends contributed to the diaper fund at the baby shower. We bought the covers with assorted snaps and Velcro that could expand as she grew, and we stocked up on the soft organic inserts.

Deja never got diaper rash, even *once*. We never needed to use the plethora of butt paste we received at the shower. The cloth diapers were definitely softer on her skin and it felt good knowing we were not contributing to the landfill.

I am not a big environmentalist, but I try to do my part. Mostly, I love to save money. The best complement to cloth diapers is by far the *Bum Genius* diaper sprayer. It's a high-pressure hose that hooks to the side of your toilet and you just spray the poop off of the diaper into the toilet and then throw the insert into the washer. It's really very simple. And it even doubles as a hose for your own bum!

After a while, the inserts become stained, but lying them in the sun helps bleach them out. After dozens of washes, you'll want to buy newer softer inserts, but it still beats the price of disposable diapers by a long shot. However, had we not had a washer and dryer, it would have required a laundry or diaper service, which would have most likely rivaled the cost of disposable diapers.

It Takes a Village

I think what saved us the most money was the community support we got from *Venice Moms*. As I mentioned, it is a local email group on Yahoo here in Los Angeles. Whenever you have questions—which are endless as a new mom—you post an email and receive back several responses from helpful loving mothers who take the time to share their wisdom and experience. As a new mom without her own mother to call on, this is *invaluable!* So many women in Los Angeles are here without parents because many of us have come here to create happier lives for ourselves, to live in a better climate or advance our careers.

With my deceased mother *not* being a phone call away, I only had a couple of aunts I could call. Since I am such an old mother, they can barely recall mothering infants themselves. Besides, things have changed and advanced so much since then.

This is why it helps to hear from local moms who have *recently* had experience with your predicament and can also guide you to a great resource nearby. I will always be grateful to this wonderful loving group of giving women.

For a new parent, when anything is wrong with your child, you will panic when you are not sure what to do. One night when Deja's hands and feet were cold, we were concerned because she typically runs hot. Before we knew about *Venice Moms*, we scoured the internet for information about what it might mean. One of the answers we found from a mom online was as simple as this: "Sometimes their hands and feet are cold. That's what socks and mittens are for." We laughed and realized we were probably getting too obsessive.

Aside from the guidance and advice from our local moms, we received many great hand-me-downs for little or next to nothing, often for free! Our first crib was free and came from a mom whose daughter had then graduated to a toddler bed. I felt that justified my investment in a brand new organic mattress. The crib lasted us until she was about two and a half years old, at which time she moved up into her own toddler bed that I got from yet another Venice Mom for the price of one massage.

Other great items we saved on were swings, bouncers, our co-sleeper, a Bumbo, baby carriers, toys, books, a toddler table and chairs, and our all-time favorite item we still use now—the bike chariot which saved us at least $400.

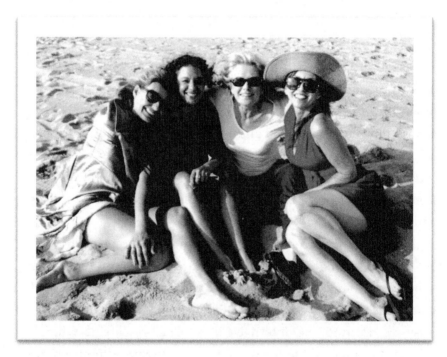

My Village of Moms Over 40 - Linda, Dana, Annie, Me

Nothing to Fear But Fear Itself

My childbirth prep class lasted for six weeks. I really enjoyed attending these meetings with the other five couples in our group. Mario was extremely supportive and enjoyed them even more than I did, probably because *I* was the one who was physically uncomfortable. It's comforting being around other women who are about to drop and pop and have all the same physical complaints.

I am about to share with you something that I believe is a game changer when it comes to pregnancy, labor, delivery and probably also applies to life in general. What my experience has led me to strongly believe is this:

It all comes down to your mindset—

what you are willing to allow in ... or block out.

I mentioned earlier that I refused to buy in to the fact that I was considered by statistics to be "high risk." I felt very healthy, so I simply blocked out that notion from my consciousness and would not allow that in at all.

Knowing I had a low pain threshold, I knew the delivery could potentially be the biggest challenge of my life, so I knew I needed to cultivate a wise inner dialogue to get through it all. Yes, the midwife and Mario would be with me, but I also knew it would be all about how I was going to think and talk myself through the process.

In one class we were given paper with paints and crayons to create a drawing of our "power animal" that were meant to help us visualize ourselves as these 'warrior mother' types to carry us through the process. Honestly, all I could think to draw was my inner Kourtney Kardashian.

I'm embarrassed to admit I know this, but when she delivered her first child (her son Mason), it was on camera and she didn't even scream. She merely reached down and pulled him out of her vagina! I don't know if she had drugs or not—my internet research is inconclusive and when it comes to reality TV, you can never be sure about what's truly factual. But while I was pregnant and watched that episode, she instantly became my new hero. Although . . . I'm *guessing* she had an epidural.

After watching *The Business of Being Born* I knew I did not want to subject my perfect new baby to the toxic chemicals of Pitocin or whatever chemicals comprise the epidural. I also didn't want that needle going into my spine. Don't get me wrong. I *love* drugs—especially painkillers. I'm the happiest girl in the world when I feel no pain. But on this day of all days, why couldn't I just grit and bear it? Millions of women had done it before me for the last 200,000 years. And hospitals have only been around for— what? 100?

My thought was, "How could it possibly be worse than your worst day of the stomach flu when it is coming out of both ends, when all you can do is continually vomit, when you are sweating profusely and you feel like you are about to die and you are on the cold tile floor begging for God to help you?"

I'm sure there are women out there who would say "it *can*," and "Yes, Liz, it's *worse!*" Even in hindsight, I still don't think it's much worse than that. You survive it. Sure, there may be pain in a whole *new* area. You might rip or tear like I did. Your 'flower' might not look as 'floral' afterward. You might be in bed resting for two weeks, but as with the stomach flu, you *do* survive it.

One of the women in my childbirth prep class had this horrible fear that something might go terribly wrong. I assumed this thought played out in her head many times if she was willing to mention it in our small group of first-time mothers and fathers.

The midwives were really great about providing the full picture on what we could expect with as many *this-could-happen* scenarios as possible. Towards the end of one of our last classes, they were listing several possible birthing scenarios, which were *awful*. This is when I decided to get up and leave. I really didn't want to expose my consciousness to these ideas. The truth is, I was too irritable and uncomfortable to sit there listening to them. With so many variables, I felt in good hands with professionals who would *know* what to do if these things happened.

All I could let into my brain were happy thoughts and positive outcomes. I was determined to expose myself strictly to people and entertainment that were either comedic or educational — no violence or drama that led to any ill feelings of any kind. I was hyper sensitive and this was no time to let myself get swept into any sort of darkness whatsoever.

Remember the woman who was afraid of something horrible happening? She did, in fact, have a long, arduous 30-hour labor with complications. This is another reason why I strongly believe that so much of what we manifest begins with our mental state.

The renowned 'guru' of midwifery, Ina May Gaskin, discusses this in a TED Talks speech you can find on YouTube. Ina May discusses a book called *Childbirth Without Fear* by Grantly Dick-Read. The main idea of the book is that unbearable labor pain is almost always associated with fear and lack of good understanding during pregnancy and perhaps a lack of understanding during labor.

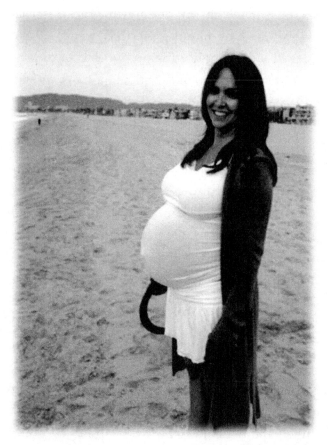

About to Drop—Marina Del Rey Peninsula 2010

She also added a profound statement:

"We are the only species that doubts its capacity to give birth."

Ina May shares some things you can do that help:

Get out of bed
Walk around
Dance
Eat something
Roll around on a ball
Doing the figure 8s
Lie on your side
Squat
Kissing your partner
Leaning forward on all fours can help open the pelvis
Pulling down on something above you, won't allow you to tighten
    up down below
Having a calm atmosphere
Dimming the lights helps because as you dilate, the pupils
    dilate — which don't like bright lights
Humor sometimes helps

Gaskin learned a lot from other cultures whose women have not succumbed to the fear (and who have perhaps *not* been exposed to American films and television which dramatize birth as a terrifying event).

Ina May Gaskin, MA, CPM, Honorary PhD, is founder and director of the *Farm Midwifery Center* in Tennessee. Early in her career she learned from indigenous midwives in Guatemala, an effective method for dealing with an obstetrical complication called Shoulder Dystocia — when babies' shoulders become stuck during birth.

This would later become known as the 'Gaskin Maneuver.' In December of 2011, Ina May received the Right Livelihood Award, also known as the Alternative Nobel Prize.

With regard to how fear affects labor, below are a few more things to consider from *The Business of Being Born*:

"In the last 40 or 50 years the medical profession convinced women that they do not know how to birth."
-Nadine Goodman, Public Health Specialist

"People think they are going to the hospital to have a safer birth, without any understanding of the subtle energies that will make their birth less safe because they are in the hospital.   Just being in an institution where fear runs around the corridors is going to impede or interfere with your labor, just being there, no matter what else they do or don't do to you. . . The place of birth has a massive effect on the kind of birth that happens.   When you are with people who trust you, your capacity for trust in yourself grows and thus your ability to give birth on your own also grows."
-Robbie Davis-Floyd, PhD MBOBB

My favorite quote from *The Business of Being Born*:

*"A woman really doesn't need to be rescued.
It's not the place
for the knight in shining armor.
It's the place for her
to face her darkest moment,
and lay claim to her victory
so that she can lay claim to her victory
after she's done it."*

-Cara Muhlhahm, Certified Nurse Midwife

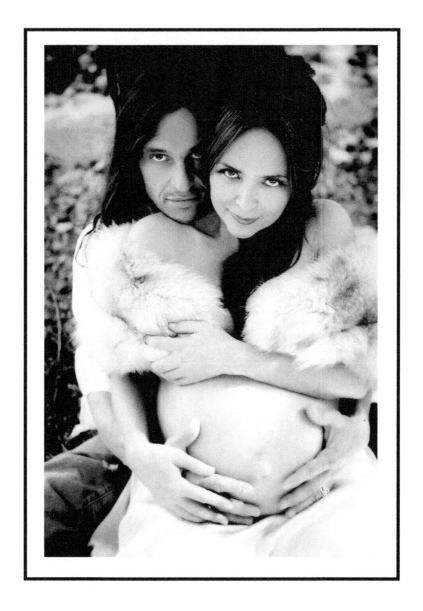

VERY Pregnant Liz and Mario - Lori Dorman Photography

ACT III

New Kid in Town

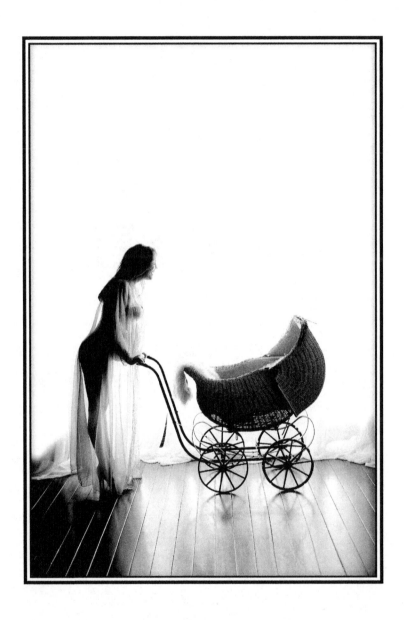

"Overdue"
Lori Dorman Photography

Deliverance!

The night before I went into labor I was already 4 days late. It was the night of my very last class at the *Sanctuary*—infant CPR. I was miserably uncomfortable so it was very hard paying attention to the information. The mere thought of having to resuscitate my newborn child was exceptionally horrifying and irritating.

As fearful as I had always been about delivering a child through my vagina, by the time baby dropped down and my due date was behind me, all I cared about was getting that baby into the light of day and onto the *other* side of my belly!

I griped and moaned my way out the door and back home to bed, hoping to get through another night without too much heartburn. The best thing I found for heartburn, by the way, was Goji Berry juice and Kefir.

It was December 20, 2010 and the next day would be my last chance to have a Sagittarius. My mother was a Sag and my being a Leo proved to be a great match for our relationship. Fire signs really understand each other. Since we never fought and got along so famously, I had hoped my daughter would also be a Sagitarrius; perhaps it might raise *our* level of compatibility.

In fact, when I first got pregnant and initially calculated what her birthday might be, it was in a dream. I actually woke myself up when I said out loud, "December 21st!" My official due date was December 16.

Another girlfriend, Linda West, who has taught me a great deal about astrology, has authored books on manifestation, is a Mayan scholar and hosts a YouTube channel called Morning

Mayan. Therefore, I had heard a lot about this date. As December 21, 2012 is the last day of the Mayan calendar, it seemed an auspicious date.

I remembered pondering the thought of it literally being the end of the world. Perhaps the ancient prophets could foresee an asteroid ending us all. I thought, "Well, if we all die, we all go together." I would only have Deja for two years.

This got me thinking about the movie *Steel Magnolias*. Julia Roberts' character was told she wasn't strong enough to carry or birth a baby. She told her mother, played by Sally Field, that she would "rather have a few minutes of wonderful than a whole lifetime of nothing special."

That same day, December 20, Mario's younger daughter, Adelina, had kicked in her sister Jasmine's bedroom door that was locked with a dead bolt. Teenagers and their clothes... enough said. She actually broke the doorjamb and it was a tattered mess with paint chips all around the floor. Mario was understandably livid. This was the last straw.

We were just about to bring a new life into the world, and more importantly our home, which should be a peaceful sanctuary. We didn't need this level of negative energy and animosity swirling about in our space.

Mario decided to take her back to her mother in Orange County. When they finally got there, Adelina was so angry she took a few swings at him and pulled his hair. She actually removed a rather large chunk from the top front of his head while he held her tightly to contain her swings. It was a sad night wracked with heavy drama. We were up all night until it was nearly morning and almost time for Mario to get up for work at 5:30 a.m.

That's when it happened; my very first contraction.

It was as if the universe was paving the road for a peaceful entry so Deja could make her big splash — her highly anticipated debut — in a calm quiet space.

I felt badly for Adelina because she was not a happy camper. Understandably, she had a lot of pent up anger that went unexpressed and unexplained. There was nothing either of us could do at that point to repair what is an inside job. That would take time. Teenagers are a special breed and cling to their emotions like air.

But as things kept happening "for a reason," on that particular day, any negative energy had suddenly been removed from the home. *Poof!* Gone...

I wasn't sure if this was another false alarm — those infamous 'Braxton Hicks' contractions always leave you doubtful about whether or not you are actually about to begin your labor. All I knew was I had been up all night and all I wanted to do was SLEEP! But the next contraction came about five minutes later. Was *this* it? Was it time?

I didn't know, but Mario had to go to work. He was working on his big project in Santa Monica Canyon, so although he was the general contractor and had many subcontractors and workers to manage, he still had the freedom to be there for me when the time came to usher Deja into our lives.

I told him not to worry. I would be fine. I *was* fine — until the next contraction came five minutes later. Then I was *not so fine*. This went on and on. They kept coming in rapid succession and were growing increasingly more intense. I don't know how many texts I sent Mario that morning telling him I was fine, and then saying, "I think I'm going into labor," only to be followed by, "Don't worry, I'm fine." "*THIS IS IT!*" Mario assumed this could go on all day, so he decided to get what he needed to get done at work and everyone there on task.

I called Annie, who lived down the block and she came right over. I wasn't sure who would be my midwife yet. Of all the midwives from the *Sanctuary*, my favorite was Racha. She was a beautiful mother of two (at the time) with beautiful mocha skin and long, groovy dreadlocks. She had come from a long line of midwives and had been present at over 1,000 births. She had the best energy, so relaxed and amusing, always laughing at Mario's stupid jokes (supplemented by foul language and sexual innuendo). Because I felt so relaxed in her presence, I prayed she would be there for my delivery.

The *Sanctuary* employed several midwives but since there were also several mommies-to-be, there were no guarantees. Racha was, in fact, available that morning and I was thrilled!

I had taken a Tylenol at this point and the pain had grown so intense that it made me nauseous and I threw it up. Annie called Racha and asked her if I could take a Vicodin. She told Annie I could go ahead and take the Vicodin, but I would probably throw that up as well. I knew I wasn't about to waste my last one — those things are golden in emergencies! So that was it. There would be no painkillers, no Tylenol, no anything.

My only source of comfort would be my team. It was indeed much like I expected, a rough day in the bathroom, as if I had the stomach flu and I was praying to God (or even the porcelain god) for help. Annie drew me a nice warm bath. She was alone with me for about the first hour before my doula showed up.

Carol Song was also my favorite acupuncturist from the Costa Acupuncture clinic. Her name is redundant, but it suits her—like a walking talking melody. She's a tiny and delicate Korean woman with the face of an angel. When I first told her I was pregnant, she told me she was becoming a doula. I asked her if she wanted to be there for my birth and she said she would be honored! She had the *most* gentle energy you can imagine, a very welcome addition to my birth team.

As I approached my due date, she recommended Moxa sticks. You can Google how to use them or search "Moxibustion." They sort of look like cigarettes that you light and hold near your baby toes. The warmth is supposed to help stimulate the acupuncture points to induce a smoother flow of blood and qi (chi) in the pelvic area and uterus, supposedly also serving to turn breech babies.

There are many great massage therapists who specialize in a type of prenatal massage that helps induce your labor. Ancient Current on YouTube accurately demonstrates how to massage pressure points to help induce as well.

Carol showed up at 8:30 a.m. She helped with acupressure during my intense contractions. Between the time Annie showed up at 7:30 and the time Mario and my midwife arrived, I had already taken 3 baths.

When you are having contractions (which I feel are the sum total of all the cramps that didn't happen over the last 9 or 10 missed periods), the most comforting place in the world is the warm water. Maybe it's a great equalizer to balance what's going on—on both sides of your belly. Once the tub water cools off, you need to empty and refill to warm it up.

When in labor, your body gives off so much heat that the whole room gets hot and the windows steam up. If someone

123

opens the door, you would think it was the tundra—frrrrrrreezing!

Somewhere in the midst of the misty-morning madness, I managed to let Mario know it was *time to come home!* By 10:30 the midwives arrived, quickly followed by Mario.

Racha brought two apprentice midwives, Heather and Heather Ann. She also came equipped with an inflatable swimming pool that would be set up in our bedroom. We moved the bed up against the wall and they filled the tub with a hose that ran from our shower. They laid out plastic sheets everywhere so it resembled a scene from *Dexter*.

This is when Mario said, "Ladies, just a warning—my shorts are coming off." The midwives all chimed in, "Yes, we know, we've been prepared for that." He quickly undressed and got into the tub with me and never left my side. For whatever reason, he wanted to be in there naked with me. Perhaps because we conceived her naked, he wanted to birth her the same way. He wrapped his legs around me and let me brace his hands during each contraction.

Carol continued using acupressure on my wrists and ankles and instructed Mario where to apply pressure as well. Racha perched herself over the side of the tub while my beloved Annie hovered about with her camera. I'm lucky to have a best friend who is a talented photographer and can effectively capture a mood and a beautiful moment (as well as the ugly painful ones).

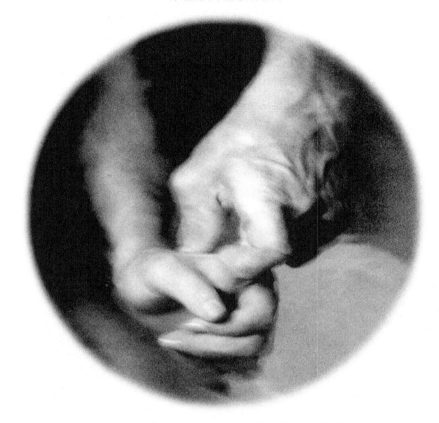

Bracing for Contractions - by *Annie Flatley*

At this point I can honestly say, I don't remember a lot. I just remember being exhausted after not having slept all night, so I basically went into a half-asleep zone between each painful contraction.

What stands out most in my mind was the mistiness of the day. Outside it was overcast and foggy. Inside, it was the same. My heat was fogging up all the windows and our bedroom was already white, with white bedding, white walls and paintings that were of the underwater palette.

I recall the hypno-birthing coach who attended one of our meetings. She told us something that I kept reminding myself through the entire labor. She explained that the fear is what will make the contractions hurt more. Much like a car accident, if you are drunk you can relax, whereas if you are sober, you are highly likely to tense up and hurt yourself more.

I paid attention to Racha as she consistently reminded me to put my shoulders down and to take deep breaths. She had this business licked for sure. The breathing part came naturally to me. I had been practicing yoga for more than ten years leading up to this, and during those moments my breathing was my only source of strength and focus.

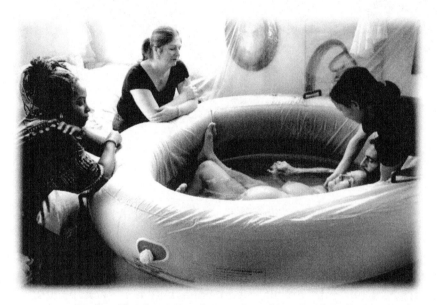

Racha, Heather, Carol, Mario and Me, Mid-Labor

At one point while one of the Heathers was leaning over the edge of the tub, Mario sees the tattoo on her chest and asks, "Is that a butterfly?" This is where most women in labor will begin to scream obscenities at her husband. I just asked in disgust, "Can we please *FOCUS?!*"

It was around this time when the most annoying point of the labor came into play. Heather went to check to see how dilated I was. *Annoying* isn't a strong enough word. But there was some good news. I strongly suspect the water must play a huge part in relaxing, expanding, and allowing you to dilate because this was the first time she checked. You may hate me for saying this but I was already 9.5 centimeters dilated. Perhaps the last 4 hours in warm water (which I refused to exit) was actually my saving grace.

Don't get me wrong. It definitely hurt pushing her out and I ripped. Her ear even got a bit stuck in the birth canal and it still sticks out to this day.

Another of the most annoying moments of my labor came when Heather checked the baby's heart rate with the doppler. It was extremely uncomfortable and I was not very happy with her at this point. I noticed she had the jobs that were making me sort of hate her, which was weird because she was so likable.

No Pain . . . No Gain

In the deepest throes of labor I screamed and squealed like a pig — sometimes like a seal, like a lion, like a monkey, like every animal in the jungle or the farm. I heard sounds come out of me so deep and guttural I didn't even know I was capable of making.

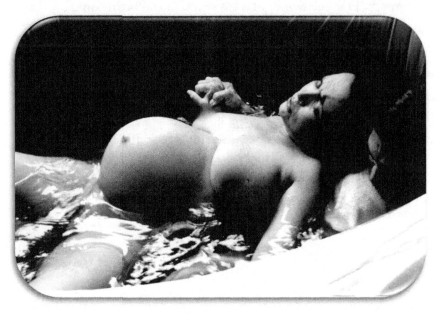

Serious Contractions

So many of my friends, especially mothers who had their babies in the hospitals, thought I was so brave. I didn't feel brave at all. I felt like a toddler who needed its blanket.

My blanket **was** *the warm water.*

At this point, Molly Ringwald is my new hero — with all of her complications and she delivered naturally, *she* wins for bravery. To me, the hospital was the scarier option. I had three experienced midwives who would know if I were truly in need of a hospital. I felt safe enough knowing the closest hospital was a short 10-minute car ride away. Had Racha told me we needed to go, I would not have hesitated.

One of my clients shared a story with me that his friend went against her midwife's plea to go to the hospital and ultimately lost her baby because she was determined to have it at home. Let this be a lesson to always trust your midwife.

In fact, our friends, Mendy and Dominic, who had their daughter a year later, were intrigued by our experience and chose the same birth plan with the *Sanctuary*. During the labor, their baby's heart rate had dropped. Their attending midwife Aleks called the paramedics immediately. Once they got to the hospital, Mendy delivered within 20 minutes and they both said they still wouldn't have chosen to do things *any* differently.

If I can leave you with anything to remember from reading this book, no matter which course of action you decide on, my best advice would be to enlist the help of a seasoned midwife. Whether you deliver at home or in the hospital and you want to *try* to do it naturally, a midwife will guide you. She will be your voice when you can't think straight and help assure you whether or not you are indeed in need of interventions. That kind of peace of mind is worth all the tea in China.

An Ideal Birth

It almost didn't happen, but I'm so happy that Carol managed to figure out my camera just in the knick of time. We were able to get the last five to ten minutes of labor on film. It's not exactly fun to watch because I'm screaming in pain. It was a bit bloody, but not too bad. I think it is slightly less ghastly if it's happening under water.

I showed the video to Deja when she turned 2 and she didn't seem bothered by it or fazed in the slightest. She was smiling and wanted to get in the water with Mommy and Papi. I assured her, "You are definitely *in* there, Deja!"

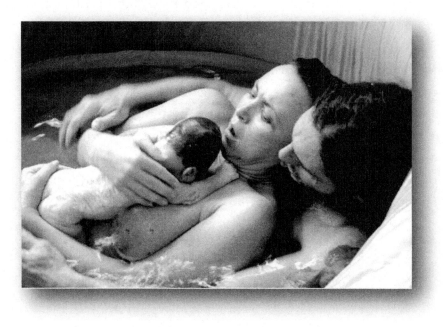

Deja Fresh from the Womb

When Deja came out, she was a dark shade of purple and covered with a thick white film called vernix. Mario wasted no time licking it off like a wild savage, or like a lion grooming its cub. But maybe he should have waited —

"Often called "Natures Cold Cream" vernix, the white creamy stuff most babies are born with, and amniotic fluid have similar immune enhancing properties as breast milk. We have known for a long time that the immunologic properties of breast milk are what truly set it apart from any other form of infant sustenance. The body of a newborn baby is very vulnerable and it does not have inborn defense mechanisms to protect itself from the environment outside of the womb. This study shows that the extremely popular procedure of "artificial rupturing of membranes" can take away the amniotic fluid's protective capability. This also holds true for bathing your baby in the first 24 hours after birth and not allowing the vernix to be absorbed into the baby's skin." — BabyCenter.com

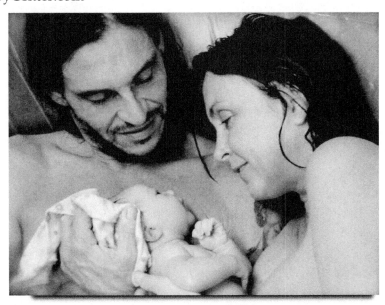

The Family Photos Begin

After a few minutes, Deja got her color and turned lighter shades of pink then finally white. Her lips that looked massive in the 4-D ultrasound were just as big in person. They were as beautiful as ever, and against her pale porcelain skin, they were bright red.

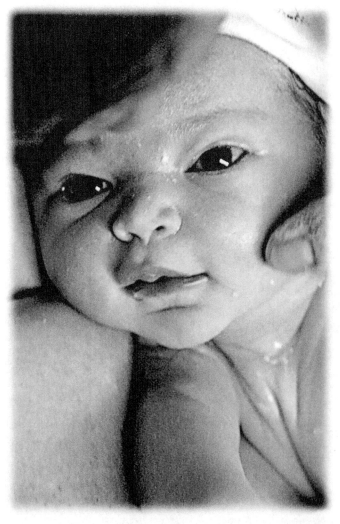

Deja Makes Her Debut

While I was pregnant, every time we had watched a water birth on film, Mario would cry and ask for a tissue gushing, "It gets me every time." Just like a punch line, he said it again when Deja appeared outside of my belly. We both held her while Annie was snapping away with the camera. We got so many great photos – 420 to be exact.

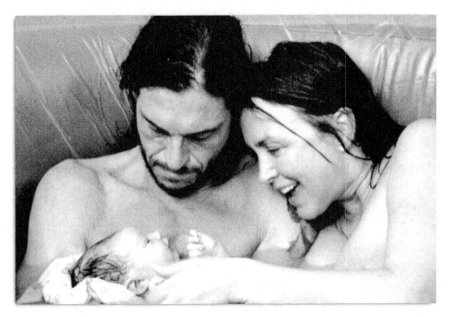

Deja meets Mommy and Papi

Having all that female energy in the room was amazing. This was especially true since my mother could not be there with me (in human form anyway). I believe she was 'there' for every priceless moment.

My doula Carol said to me, "You just had my *ideal* birth!" I would think so, since she had only been there for four hours. I'm embarrassed to admit that on video I actually responded, "Well, I'm glad it was ideal for you. All I know is my pussy is KILLING me!" Really, Liz? Did you have to use that word of all the words to describe the female anatomy? You can't use any other word—like vag, cooch, flower, cookie, hooha, anything else? Nope! On video you have to use the one word that makes you sound like some kind of porn actress. Great.

When Deja first came out, they laid her on me and I couldn't believe what was happening. Now that she was finally out, oh YES! I have this human I'm responsible for now... What will she want first? To see everything! She opened her eyes and looked around, looking deeply into everyone's eyes. Deja was wide awake, totally alert and just as curious that first day as she has been every day since.

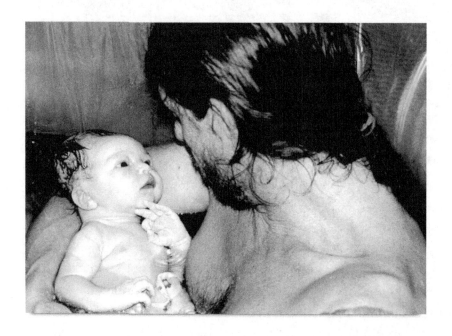

Deja Lets Papi Know she is "Okay"

The total labor lasted just a little over 7 hours. SUCCESS! Time of birth: 12:51 p.m., 12.21.2010. It's a bit eerie that I had predicted this date just 9 months prior.

When Annie told a friend about Deja's birth, she said, "What? Annie, you know that means she is a star child!" We know that 12.21.2012 is the end of the Mayan Calendar. Evidently two years prior to the end of the Mayan Calendar, the very day of the birth was supposedly greatly revered by spiritual leaders around the world. I'm suspecting because it was both the winter solstice *and* the lunar eclipse. It is said that a huge portal opened on that day that supposedly brought to Earth a massive amount of cosmic energy. I can't attest to that personally, but I can tell you that *my* huge portal opened that day, letting *out* a huge amount of cosmic energy.

I think it took another 20-30 minutes before the placenta was expelled. Once I was finally free of it and they cut the cord, I jumped out of the tub, went to the bathroom and immediately into *my* shower. Having my body back to myself with the labor pains behind me, that first shower was euphoric. Immediately following such an ordeal, my own shower was *exactly* where I wanted to be. My eyes were finally wide open, as if I were finally awake for the first time all day.

While I was showering, Mario was in another world altogether. He stayed in the tub holding and examining Deja for a long time and didn't care about the blood in the tub or the placenta floating in the bowl. He was a trooper when it came to anything gross. I loved him for that. I think they bonded deeply during that time because she is definitely "Papi's little girl."

During my pregnancy, Mario would always nuzzle up to my belly and speak to Deja in Spanish very lovingly. So when Racha was doing the neurological tests on her and she was fussing, he nuzzled up to her ear and said all the things he would say to her when she was in the womb. It instantly quieted her down. To this day, he wakes her with multiple soft kisses and loving words. She is putty in his hands...*siempre.*

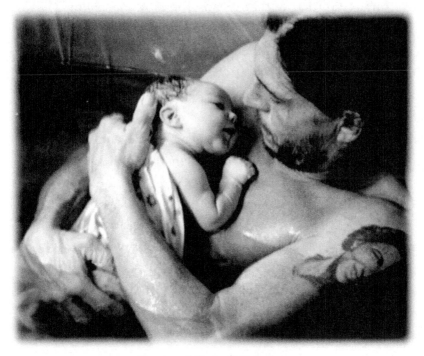

Papi and Deja Fall in Love

Placenta Power

One of my favorite perks of having the midwives manage our birth was their service of freeze-drying and encapsulating the placenta. Jacqueline, the midwife who led our childbirth prep classes did the deed. She told me I had a "beautiful juicy placenta." Well, now *there's* a compliment you don't hear every day.

Once encapsulated, you can simply ingest it as a supplement, like vitamins. If someone handed you a jar of placenta capsules, you would never be the wiser. I find nothing gross about that.

On the other hand, when I was a teenager I heard a story from a girlfriend that scarred me for life. It's one of those stories you can't un-hear or erase from your memory. Her parents had friends over for dinner whose dinner conversation included the fact that they ate their placenta by sautéing it with chicken. Now *that* sounded disgusting.

In truth, the health benefits of ingesting placenta are phenomenal for the mother and her newborn. It is said that it helps with the postpartum depression as well as assisting the milk production. I've also read that it is the most nutrient-rich supplement you can put in your body. The cost of having the placenta encapsulated was around $300 and well worth the piece of mind, knowing it had so many incredible benefits. Jasmine took one, and then post-epiphany, sighed, "Oh God. I just ate a piece of *Liz*."

All grossness aside, I can attest to the fact that, perhaps due to the placenta pills, I experienced zero postpartum depression and I had no problem producing milk. I was practically a cow dressed as a milkmaid with my own personal dairy. My milkshake definitely brought Mario to the yard. My real problems didn't surface until about the second week of breastfeeding.

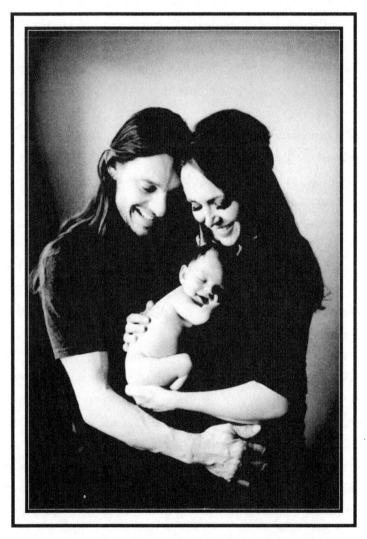

2-week-old family - Lori Dorman Photography

Peace at Last

About 30 minutes after the birth, Jasmine came home with her friend Emilie. They were bewildered by the silence in the house. All was quiet and peaceful, even though there were now ten people in the house and Mario and I were still in the water with Deja. Everyone was mesmerized by this new life that had us all transfixed.

After my luxurious post-labor shower, Mario was *still* in the tub, entranced by his new daughter. So I jumped back in with them while Annie shot more photos of our family.

Mario always loves to tell the story of how I got out of the tub, went onto the bed and immediately asked for my laptop so I could post the birth on Facebook. He thought that was insane. I had been inundated with texts since my due date, everyone asking if I had the baby yet, so I felt it was the fastest way to inform everyone she had finally arrived without having to send out dozens of texts.

A total of 14 people held Deja on her first day on earth. Other friends stopped by. Our whole family ate ice cream in bed. Even though Jasmine was angry about her bedroom door getting kicked in, she was so sad that her sister Adelina went home to her mom and we were all disappointed that she *just* missed the birth of her new sister. She also sadly missed the first six months of Deja's life. On the bright side, Deja now had a bedroom of her own and there was peace in the house. It was a truly wonderful day and the beginning of a spectacular life.

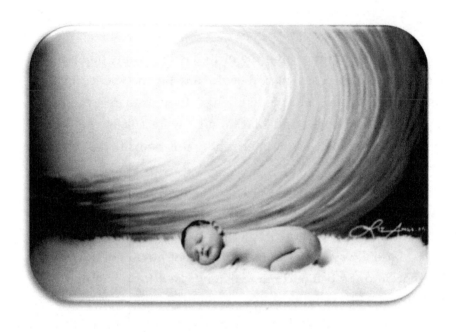

Deja with 'Wave' *by Liz Angeles*
Lori Dorman Photography

Riding the Wave

In *More Business of Being Born/Special Deliveries: Celebrity Mothers Talk Straight on Birth*, Melissa Joan Hart was so anxious to get her baby out, that she asked the doctor to induce her, and that Pitocin caused so many complications that at one point, she had 9 things attached to her body. She thinks her son wasn't ready and probably would have stayed in there another two weeks. She added that everything about it felt phony, not right and not *real*.

Cindy Crawford explains that without all the hospital distractions, a new environment and strange people, you go inward more and tune in more to your inner dialogue. I agree. I know I would not have been so focused or fearless had I been in a place of fear (in a place *I* fear; the hospital).

Gisele Bundchen explains that being at home with your mom, your husband, your midwife, your music, etc. makes you feel safe. I could not agree more. I feel that is what makes things go easier, if it makes you feel more relaxed, as long as you are trusting in yourself and your team.

Cindy and Gisele both described their births like the power of the ocean forming an internal wave. You can either fight it, which will slam you down, or you can dive into the wave and ride it. That concept could not have been more aptly described — at least with regard to *my* experience of really feeling the entire labor.

Compromising Situations

If the thought of being at home and not close enough to a hospital to feel truly safe, you might want to consider a hospital birth center (HBC).

HBCs can be a great option that marries both benefits. They are typically in a separate wing or on another floor within the hospital. They are often equipped with a double bed for the couple, a hot tub, and the emergency equipment is tucked away so that you don't have the medical vibe in your periphery.

Staffed primarily by midwives who are experienced in dealing with natural births, it can be a great option for husbands who say "No way!" to the idea of a home birth. The best thing about HBCs is that you don't enter through hospital doors, which can be a scary place, often slowing down or stopping the labor. However, the hospital protocols will still apply. If you are in labor for more than 24 hours, they will strongly urge you to induce, which will quite often result in C-section.

"If you're on a floor where anesthesia is accessible, usually the epidural rate goes up to 90% very quickly. Clinicians have a comfort zone with what they are used to."
-Richard Jennings, CNM, MBOBB

On the other hand, freestanding birth centers are *not* connected to a hospital. Historically, hospitals are where people go when they are sick and dying, so when birthing women go to hospitals and go through the door, they often become fearful.

That fear and the resulting stress and anxiety are what can slow down or stop the labor.

Aleksandra Evanguelidi, LM, CPM, Co-clinical Director for Midwifery Services at *Sanctuary Birth Center*, was one of the midwives who counseled me during my pregnancy. Aleks was my midwife who drove the point home, that was my internal mantra throughout my labor:

"Your body was designed for this."

In *MBOBB*, Aleks was interviewed by Ricki Lake at the *Sanctuary*, the only freestanding birth center in Los Angeles *at the time* of the filming.

As I write this in 2014, there are currently six free-standing birth centers. It appears that what I am told may hold some truth—midwifery, natural birth and home birth are all trending back!

The *Sanctuary* wanted to give people the option to have the sense they could really relax in a sort of home away from home. In their birth center, they use candles, dimmers, sheets with high thread count, an organic mattress, etc. They also have a back-up doctor available who works at Cedars Sinai Hospital. When they transport, your care plan is on file. She says that out of 1,000 women, maybe five may have an emergency transport.

*"When you don't push past a woman's natural rhythms you're not going to have the body doing really weird things. You really need to step into your primal body when you are delivering because those are all hormones that are going to kick in when you are in that mammalian experience - you are going to need to use to get down into it. **Wherever you feel the safest is where you need to be**. So for some women it is the*

hospital. For other people, it's at home in the bedroom, even often in the bathroom."

-Aleksandra Evanguelidi, MBOBB

I have just learned that the *Sanctuary* has announced it will be closing its doors this year. I am saddened by this news because I am so grateful for my experience under their care. However, since our time with the *Sanctuary*, one of the new freestanding birth centers was founded by our cherished midwife Racha Lawler who opened *The Community Birth Center* in Los Angeles.

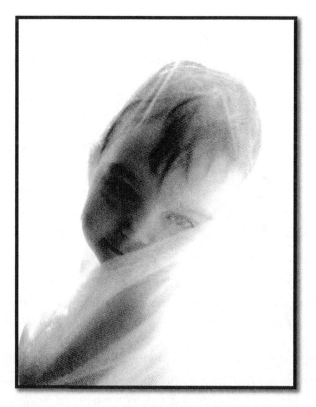

Our Bundle

The Cost of Being Born

A study was performed by the University of California, San Francisco.

"The study found that California women giving birth were charged from $3,296 to $37,227 for an uncomplicated vaginal delivery, depending on which hospital they visited. For a C-section, women were billed between $8,312 and nearly $71,000. Few of the women in the study had serious health issues and most were discharged within six days of admission."

-UCSF.EDU

Probably the biggest downside of natural home birth and midwifery care is the fact that insurance does not cover it. How tragic is that? In the event of a hospital birth, which I had hoped to avoid, I was fortunate to be covered by AIM (Access for Infants and Mothers) by the State of California *www.aim.ca.gov* -- for only $500. I have no idea how much that would have covered or how much more it might have cost had we needed hospital services. It can go in so many different directions.

Since we didn't need to use that, our cost in 2010 for prenatal care, midwifery care, childbirth education and preparation, lactation classes, coaching, delivery and postpartum care totaled out at $6,500.

I was so fortunate and grateful that Mario could cut one check mid-pregnancy, and we never received another invoice again. Had he not been in that financial position at the time, I would not have had access to this level of ancient wisdom, motherly support and tender loving care.

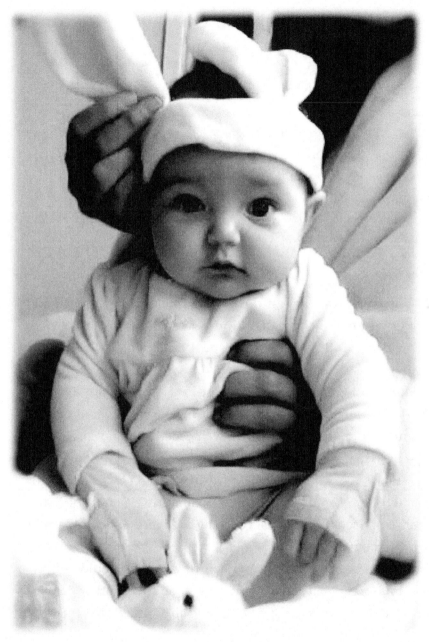

Deja Bunny – 3 Months

Nursing 101

I feel that breastfeeding is by far the most painful part of the mothering process. It's not just the day you are delivering. It's every day, day after day, over and over again, and it *hurts!* Granted, Deja had no trouble latching and I had no trouble with my milk production, but the truth is I have always had sensitive nipples. Yes, this goes hand in hand with my "hyper-sensitivity" but having your nipples fondled or licked as opposed to bitten is one story.

It's quite another story to have a professional nipple sucker putting their 'palette pedal' to the metal and sucking mercilessly on those puppies for hours upon hours, day after day. After the first week to ten days, I think I was just about raw. It's as though my nipples had transformed into nothing more than mere scabs.

I had heard so many great benefits about immunity building that comes from nursing and had personally witnessed its benefits and lack thereof, from its absence. I was told by a woman that when I was born in the mid 60s, it wasn't "fashionable" to breast feed. Women's lib was all the rage, and feeding babies formula had become standard procedure for moms of that era. They were actually told by their doctors it was superior to breast milk. Women like my mother were either brainwashed into thinking the latest and greatest was better than the boob, or more likely they were just too busy working to be bothered.

Because my immunity *sucks*, I am a firm believer that nothing beats the boob. I probably caught a cold three to four times a year before I had a baby. Now that she is in preschool, I probably average about six to seven colds a year, thanks to all of the marvelous germs she brings home. Mario was breastfed, as were his siblings, as well as his other two daughters. Whenever they get sick, they all get over it in about a day or two—whereas my colds last several days to a week.

When Deja was born and went straight for the boob with no trouble latching, I thought, "Well, this is a breeze. I have this licked! Not a problem. *Next!*"

But after that first 7-10 days

when nursing became too painful to bear,

I ate my words.

I cried and cried for hours.

I had been breastfeeding exclusively and had hoped to do that for an entire year. If I could just go a year, I would be SO happy. But here I was, a blubbering mess, up all night in tears. Mario was bewildered. He felt so helpless and had no idea what to do for me. That's when we called in the big guns.

Kimberly, the woman from the *Sanctuary* who led our breastfeeding class was a lactation coach. She offered to make a house call to help me figure things out. She asked if I had *Lansinoh* (a nipple ointment for sore cracked nipples) and I said, "Yes, but it's not helping." She asked if I had a nipple guard. "A what?" I had never even heard of one. She said she would bring one and we could discuss my nursing positions.

Kimberly had already had five children of her own, so she was clearly a pro. She told me how valuable breast milk is, and that everyone in her house uses it because it's the best thing for any cuts, scrapes, burns—you name it. She leaves her freezer stocked up with an abundance of it. You can even drop it in your baby's eyes if they have conjunctivitis.

I think the best thing that happened to me as a new mom was when Kimberly brought me that nipple guard.

It's a little plastic nipple shield with tiny holes that you place over your nipple. It gives your nipples a break from the harsh suckling and allows your baby to still get milk. This is when I discovered breast milk's miraculous healing powers. The 'breast milk bath' my nipples got between my nipple and the shield was what actually allowed my raw nipples to heal! Why had no one ever even mentioned this to me?! Within two or three days of using it, I was completely healed and never had a problem nursing again.

I managed to reach my goal and exceed it. This was a miracle for me, because I'm terrible at setting goals, let alone reaching them. Many of my veteran mommy friends told me that it would be harder for me to stop nursing than it would be for my baby. Considering what a demanding whiner Deja can be (like her mom), I seriously doubted that prospect... until I reached a year. I couldn't have known then how special those moments were, and that even though they were often annoying, they were incredibly relaxing.

After Kimberly had taught me the football position (holding her like a football), where I could nurse her as I lay on my side, I could fall asleep with Deja on me.

Nursing literally sucks the life out of you. I often joked to Mario, "I am springing forth life into our child!" Whenever she was fussy, it would instantly calm her, and we could both end in a nap.

Men just don't get it. They think all we are doing all day is getting suckled while they are hard at work. We nurse about 10-12 times a day. Do you think *any* man could be worth a damn if they expelled their bodily fluids ten times a day? They would be sleeping the rest of the day if that were the case and never get a single thing accomplished!

When all was said and done, I nursed for 18 months. I felt really good about that period of time. By the end, she still wasn't sleeping through the night and my brain was all twisted up from never having a full night's sleep. Aside from that, her teeth were getting sharp!

Here is the crazy part, and maybe yet another 'divine intervention' at play: Deja lost her first two teeth before she was a year old. They were the bottom two middle teeth.

One day, Mario was out walking her in the stroller so that I could have a break. When I heard them enter the front door from the living room, I heard huffing and puffing. I said, "What's going on?" He said, "She's *OKAY!*" Startled, I asked, "What have you done with our child?"

He liked to be playful with her and had her lap belt strapped, but not the shoulder straps, so when they strolled over one of those messed up sidewalks where the tree roots are practically exploding, she hit her head on the hand bar and instantly popped her teeth right out.

Mario thought he saw them and tried to get them out, not that it would have mattered. Deja immediately swallowed them as Mario licked all the blood off her face so she never knew anything happened. Shortly after this little incident, I called my friends and asked who could help me put an end to Mario and dispose of the body.

The dentist said it was a clean break. These days, all the kids in her class have all their teeth. When people meet Deja now, they quickly assume the tooth fairy has already visited her, but no, not the case at all.

Ultimately, what I believe happened was the universe once again conspiring in my favor, as well as Deja's. They say everything happens for a reason, right? Had those teeth been there the whole time, I am quite certain I could not have lasted for 18 months, and perhaps she would not have the strong immunity she has today. That little divot that was created from those missing teeth left just enough room for my nipple to *not* get mangled.

That was yet another lesson for me in life to understand *why* things happen. Much to our chagrin, we can't comprehend life's gifts that are in disguise as downers—until much later. Sure, she won't get her permanent teeth for a few more years and may not even be able to whistle, but you really can't put a price tag on strong immunity. Now when people ask where her teeth went, we tell them, "That's where the straw goes."

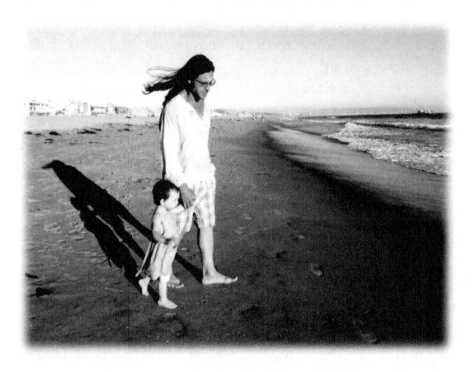

Father Daughter Beach Stroll at Sunset, 2012

Warrior Mama

One of my regular massage clients, Alexis, had two boys and sort of always wanted a girl but had no intention of having another child. One night while I was pregnant, I massaged her and she confessed to me that she missed the feeling she got from the delivery — it empowered her and made her feel like a warrior.

I laughed so hard. I could think of so many ways I could empower myself, or methods to feel like a warrior that didn't involve that kind of full-blown bodily torture. Interestingly, within about a year of that time, she and her husband were surprised with a pregnancy and she now has that baby sister for her 7 and 8-year-old boys.

Now that I have had that experience, especially having done it naturally and at home, I really *do* understand that feeling. You really *are* a warrior. It really *is* a rite of passage. Nothing will ever make me feel more proud. No accomplishment will ever surpass this.

Sure, I painted a lot of paintings while I was in my *looks-like-I'm-never-going-to-have-a-baby-so-I-may-as-well-create-something-I-can-leave-behind* phase. I had no legacy and now I do. She will be my greatest creation and my ultimate masterpiece. I can walk through life now, knowing that I'm not solely existing, taking up space.

Admittedly, I had a super groovy bevvy of female friends whose lifestyles reminded me that I could still be happy and fulfilled without a child. Still, I spent many years with the feeling that maybe it wasn't happening because I was inept, incompetent, or just made too many poor choices.

Now I feel my life has more purpose, more meaning, and the choices I make matter tremendously.

As a single woman, I could go sky diving and if I died, oh well. But now I think differently. Does it mean my life will be less risky and exciting? Probably for me personally, but who knows how things will turn out?

There are things we don't do in life because of our children or our parents. Skydiving was one of the things my mom made me promise not to do until she died. I had to respect her wishes. Her only other requests were to *not* get a tattoo or pose in Playboy (as if anyone is asking). I got my tattoo less than a year after she died, a Chinese symbol for courage — or so I *thought!*

Just last year in a yoga class, a Chinese woman asked if I knew what my tattoo meant. I said, "Uhhh, well I sure hope it means courage!" She said, "Well, sort of." "Oh no!" I said, "What *does* it mean?" She said it's actually two words and it literally means "Elite Hero." "Great!" I said. How embarrassing. She quickly comforted me by saying, "Well, if you think about it, you need to have courage to be an elite hero."

Let this be a warning to research any tattoos if they aren't in your native language. Maybe it should have been the title of my book: Elite Hero? Maybe not.

Grand Mama?

Now the problem that comes into play is being so much older than my daughter. I am an older mom and by nature, very tired. Laura Drago, my incredible acupuncturist in Mar Vista, told me I technically had a 'geriatric pregnancy.' So it is no surprise to her that I have been perpetually exhausted for the last three years.

To make matters worse, I have now entered pre-menopause and my daughter isn't even in kindergarten. Could life be any less fair to women? Those "warrior" (or *elite hero*) feelings come and go.

There may be multiple factors contributing to my exhaustion, but the fact remains, I am pushing 50 and Deja is still in preschool. I am literally a MAM (middle-aged mom). I am in bed by 9 p.m. and awake by 5 a.m. thanks to my bladder.

When she is a teenager, she may have it so easy. Will sneaking out of the house be a breeze? Will I be dead asleep or perhaps pretending to be so I don't have to fight with her? Will I be waking up as she is sneaking back in? Or will I never sleep again once she hits 13? By then I will be almost 60.

Will people be asking her if I am her grandmother? Will I be too pooped to deal with the drama or will *I* be sneaking out of the house?

I don't know what will happen, but we all learn as we go. All we can do is try to bring her up with the best values we can instill, and hope she makes the best decisions for her highest good.

My prayer is for the universe to deliver some technological or scientific breakthrough that will bless me with youthful looks and more importantly *vitality!* In the meantime, I'm open to learning any tips or tricks to feel younger, generate more energy, or any methods to increase my longevity so I can be the best mother I can to this child without dropping the ball. So please feel free to send them my way. Meanwhile, I will only be getting older by the day. Can someone please hand me my walker?

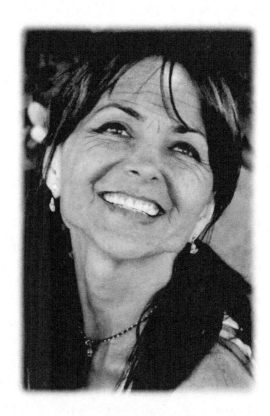

25 years from now?

Bouncing Back

Once Deja was free from my belly and I was free from bed rest, I could finally work to get my body back. Yes, I live in L.A. but luckily, I am no longer modeling or acting so I didn't particularly feel the Hollywood pressure to look fabulous.

We took long slow walks together while I was still trying to heal my torn up birth canal. Each day we would walk a little more. I decided to take it easy and didn't stress myself out about losing my baby weight. No one needs that stress, or any stress for that matter. I enthusiastically took the advice from the midwives to enjoy my 'baby moon' without feeling like I needed to look better, do more laundry, clean more, or push myself any harder than absolutely necessary.

When I did join a gym once Deja was 3 months old, it was such a relief! The Kids Club at Equinox in Santa Monica could watch her while I walked on the treadmill or reveled in the relaxing joys of yoga. I was elated to have even just a couple of hours to myself, but even more thrilled when I went back to get her and they told me what a good and easy baby she was.

I was just starting to get back to work. I was hoping all that nursing would help me lose the weight. They say it can help you burn 500-650 calories per day. It took me a while to take the weight off. I was 45 at that point and had never put on weight like that in my life. I could take off 5 or 10 pounds again and again throughout my life... but this was a new 50 pounds of flab to shed in the grueling months ahead.

Mario then informed me that if I did cardio first thing in the morning on an empty stomach, it would burn the fat off the fastest. He is not a fitness expert or personal trainer but I think that might have been his vocation were it not for his extreme passion for construction. His body rivals those of men half his age and he is now over 50.

He explains, "Your body has been at rest for about 8 hours without eating anything and the last meal that was put in the body has been digested and the nutrients taken out, the fat and leftover waste has dispersed as the body sees fit. So when you get up in the morning, your stomach, your blood stream and your system are empty. If you do 45 minutes minimum to an hour of cardio in the morning before you put *anything* in your mouth (even water) the way the body works, is it goes to the simplest food source for energy first, meaning the stomach. If there is nothing in the stomach, it will go to the blood stream to get any sugar or sucrose that might be in there. When there is nothing in there, it will go to the last source, which is the fat storage and use that fat for the energy. That will be the body's fuel and thereby burn off the fat."

How was this the first time I had learned this technique? All those formative years teaching aerobics, taking dance classes, all the gym time that created my model body in my early 20's, strenuously exercising for several hours every day — I'm just *now* learning this at 45?

I am thrilled to inform you that this method *really* works! I am not a maniac at this stage in my life, so I'm sure it could have happened much faster if I were more diligent about my diet. I did, however, successfully take the weight off slowly and safely, about a pound a week.

I'm not going to say I didn't have my moments of self-loathing and disgust. You go through so many hormonal changes and weird feelings after having a baby. You are delighted to have your body back to yourself, but your nursing baby is still your "ball and chain" that tends to weigh you down, keeps you around the house and slows you down.

It took me a good year to get back to feeling normal, but the fat indeed burned off just as Mario assured me it would. Aside from the nipple guard, that is one of the most useful pieces of information I have received in my lifetime.

I really loved hot yoga classes, but my acupuncturist Laura vehemently advised me against them. She explained that for aging women, it depletes a woman's organs of essential fluids and heat. We start producing testosterone as we age, whereas men start producing estrogen. Where is the JUSTICE? This is why their skin gets softer and they age better, while our skin gets drier. Hence, we need all the fluids we can get—and keep.

My most recent mission was to embark on *Pure Barre* classes.

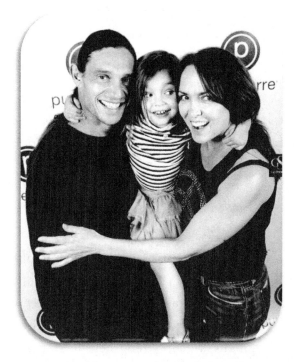

Grand Opening, Pure Barre Santa Monica 2014

Once I had attended 8 classes, I did see a very noticeable difference. My muffin top was finally shrinking down to size. Pure Barre is a series of tiny isometric exercises, using resistance bands, hand weights, small exercise balls and the ballet barre. Ladies, it *works!* Just prepare to be sore... Very sore. Alternating with yoga classes was the only way I survived it.

When it comes to losing weight, I did have great success with Dr. Schulze's Formula 1 and Formula 2. It's a simple bowel cleanse that really helps you move out any intestinal build up. It actually helped me lose almost ten pounds in about a month.

With regard to energy, I recently got a big boost from Garden of Life's Vitamin Code as well as Radiant Greens by Dr. Tony O'Donnell.

Another quick easy longevity booster that I *love* only takes me ten minutes a day. The Five Tibetan Rites are 5 yoga exercises you do — ideally 21 times each. Many people have demonstrated them on YouTube and this is what Wikipedia has to say:

"(There are) seven spinning, "psychic vortexes" within the body: two of these are in the brain, one at the base of the throat, one on the right side of the body in the vicinity of the liver, one in the reproductive anatomy, and one in each knee. As we grow older, the spin rate of the vortexes diminishes, resulting in "ill-health". However, the spin rate of these vortexes can be restored by performing the Five Rites daily, resulting in improved health."

If I had my choice, my preferred method to flatten my tummy would be Pilates. I love it because it works all the tiny muscles and seems to have the fastest results. Just when you start feeling fatigued, it's time to switch to the next exercise. Joseph Pilates created it originally to help strengthen the dancer's core. I often feel that yoga doesn't focus enough on the core, which is

160

your power source. You need a strong back to deal with a toddler's tantrums and for all the bending over you have to do to clean up toys left everywhere. I prefer the group classes since they are cheaper than private classes, but I have trouble with the scheduling. If you have the same problem or can't afford a studio, many people teach Mat Pilates on YouTube.

Last year while trying to rush Deja to school she was fighting me when I was trying to strap her into the car seat. Those toddlers are strong when they don't get their way. I was very stressed and ended up throwing out my neck and back. I suffered in pain for several months, wishing I had previously done more to strengthen my back muscles. Then, during the summer while editing this book, I spent too much time on my couch writing on my laptop and did more damage to my back until I could barely move or even bend over to wash my face. What saved my life was the three visits a week to my beloved Chiropractor Dr. Brandon Takahashi in West Los Angeles.

Once I was mostly out of the woods, I discovered the joys of Rolfing — also known as Structural Integration or Hellerwork. Instead of working your body from the outside in, it works from the inside out. I was referred to a master in his field, Dan Bienenfeld in Pacific Palisades. Every time I leave his office, I float away with no pain or discomfort — like a happy fairy. By the way, Dan told me about a woman he knows who got pregnant and had a healthy baby at 54. She makes me sound like a spring chicken!

Between the chiropractic treatments and the Rolfing, I am feeling better than I have in over a year. Another practitioner who was extremely helpful when I suffered from sciatica during my pregnancy is Neuromuscular Therapist Gadi Kaufman of Santa Monica, also known as "The Nerve Whisperer." With all the body goes through during pregnancy and the early stages of motherhood, I believe most mothers can greatly benefit from these practices.

My latest and favorite new health tip is called "Oil Pulling." It's an ancient Ayurvedic medicine practice where you take organic virgin coconut oil or sesame oil or sunflower oil, and swish it around in your mouth on an empty stomach for 15-20 minutes. Then you spit and rinse again with warm salt water. It "pulls" out all the impurities, toxins, bacteria, decay—not just from your mouth, but your body as well. People have reported this practice healed their asthma, allergies, arthritis, diabetes, PMS, migraines—all sorts of ailments.

As I mentioned, I believe I have poor immunity because I was not personally breastfed. This past fall we noticed a good long run of no colds brought home from school. Then Deja caught a cold that lingered for 10 days. Mario finally caught it and I did *not*. I was even drinking from her cups and eating off her fork. The only thing I have been doing different is 'pulling oil' daily for the past few months. I think it is really helping me because I am feeling a lot better in general. My skin looks better and my dentist even noticed a drastic difference in my gums.

It's funny how the universe brings you things when you ask for them or just write them down. Earlier I mentioned wanting to find ways to increase my vitality and longevity. Then last week I massaged a client who gave me such an education on the macrobiotic diet and lifestyle, I felt like I really should have paid *him*. He told me that when he removed things from his son's diet like chicken, eggs, pizza and dairy, he became much more patient within just two weeks. He explained that chickens have erratic energy, which we consume and absorb energetically. Although chicken and eggs are such staples in our menu, it's definitely worth a shot for results like those.

Macrobiotics means "life according to the largest view," but has also been defined as "the universal way of health and longevity." I am now learning a great deal from Denny Waxman's *The Complete Macrobiotic Diet – 7 Steps to Feel Fabulous, Look Vibrant, & Think Clearly.*

What I found to be most interesting were the testimonials. One gentleman who was coming back from chemo and radiation was able to optimize his health and impregnate his wife. Another woman who got her body on track with macrobiotics was able to conceive at 44 and then again at 51.

I am learning we should not consume foods that are not indigenous to our climate, like tropical fruits such as bananas or coconuts (unless we live in the tropics). We should have a grain and vegetable with each meal. We should take the time (he recommends 20 minutes) to have a meal while sitting, chewing our food thoroughly (25-50 times) and *not* watching TV or reading while eating.

Some of these bad habits are very challenging for me to change, but I'm determined to try. What I loved about his approach is he doesn't recommend depriving ourselves as much as he recommends *adding* things, which will in turn help our bodies crave more of the good and less of what isn't serving us.

With regard to trying to remain attractive, getting eyelash extensions has to be my all-time favorite beauty tip. Latisse is not recommended if you are pregnant or nursing, so extensions are a great alternative, just costly to maintain. They make me look and feel so much prettier. When we age, our face seems to shrink up and disappear. For me, it's the difference between walking by a mirror and feeling like, "uggh," or seeing yourself and thinking, "Hey baby, come to mama!"

Ninja Mama

When Deja turned about 5 or 6 months old, she was ready for solid foods. One of my favorite things I enjoyed doing for my deliciously happy baby was making her baby food from scratch. This is another accomplishment of which I am very proud. Sure, we bought baby food from Whole Foods at times so we would always have plenty on hand, but obviously you can't trust anything more than what you bring to the table and prepare yourself. Sometimes I even chewed up food and fed it to her from my mouth like a bird does.

The best possible thing I could think to do was go to Farmer's Market for the freshest organic ingredients available free from pesticides. With all the talk about GMOs and Monsanto these days, it's becoming blatantly clear it's our safest course of action.

We purchased the *Baby Bullet*—a blender for baby food that also comes with several trays and jars for storage. I felt this was an excellent investment because we used it daily for at least two years before it finally gave out. I still use all the little smiley-faced jars and cups, and they make me happy.

Some great tips I've learned from other health conscious moms: Put ground up green veggies in the tomato sauce that goes into pizza and pasta for unsuspecting children. Puree cauliflower and carrots into macaroni and cheese.

Jasmine learned from another mom that her kids loved vegetables because she started them on veggies *first*, at least a couple of months before she introduced fruit. I thought this was *genius*! So naturally, I followed that plan.

I made Deja's baby food out of steamed carrots, broccoli, zucchini, squash, red beets, orange beets, potatoes, purple potatoes, all the while trying to remember to feed her a rainbow every day. To this day, Deja will go to a party and will honestly choose to eat the carrots and broccoli off the food trays. One of her favorites is avocado, which is actually one of the best whole foods you can feed a baby. If I cut off the top of one, she will eat the entire avocado with a spoon.

I later introduced strawberries and bananas, cantaloupe and pineapple. Naturally, she has had every other fruit like apples, oranges, kiwis, mangos, blackberries, blueberries and raspberries. But at this point, aside from strawberries she won't eat any other berries whether solo or in oatmeal or yogurt. I therefore address all eating concerns at this point with my 'ninja-mama' philosophy.

I have the Ninja brand mixer and I make a lot of smoothies. Sometimes I will put all those berries she won't eat in her smoothies and sometimes make them into popsicles. Often times I will include protein powder or even the veggies she didn't finish the night before. Ultimately, that popsicle becomes a meal replacement. Whenever she resists my requests to do something that I really need her to do, she will jump at the chance to get a popsicle and gleefully do *anything* I ask.

I also love to make her banana ice cream out of nothing more than frozen bananas and a bit of almond milk. She thinks she is getting a treat and 'ninja-mommy' is *winning the war*! Another good recipe for a chocolate shake is fresh spinach with frozen banana, pineapple, blueberries, yogurt and cocoa powder – *Booy*ah!

Nobody's Perfect

I can't lie. It's not like Deja is a pure organic, vegan baby. I let her have little tiny lollipops now and then or a cookie here and there, and I try not to come unglued when Mario lets her have a donut. What can you do if you have to take your kids to birthday parties where every child there is eating cake? Unless your child is lactose intolerant or has Celiac disease, let them have cake!

There are some delicious recipes on-line for vegan, gluten-free and sugar free cakes and cookies, so you can experiment if you are really concerned. It's never a bad idea to help educate your own circle of concerned mothers.

When Deja was still on the boob and on solid foods, maybe around 7-8 months old, we had a date night and our resident teenage sitters had given her rice milk. Deja was a complete hyper spaz. It freaked them out. They couldn't believe it. She was babbling like she was on speed.

That's when I impressed upon the entire family: studies have shown that sugar is like meth for babies. Upon discovering the high sugar content in rice milk, we discovered that almond milk, hemp milk and coconut milk are clearly superior choices. Deja had been so pure up to this point, that too much sugar significantly affected her, and still does to this day.

In fact, if I leave her with a mom who takes her kids to McDonald's, she will come home a different person. She sort of becomes the 'Tasmanian Devil.' It's a bit scary and borderline creepy. I grew up on McDonald's, but even their standards have changed over the years.

It's no secret there is a lot of controversy over sugar now, a lot in the news about high-fructose corn syrup, gluten, and the resulting obesity in children. I grew up on a *ton* of sugar. As a child, I was always a twig with high metabolism so I was never concerned with my diet until my teens when I started to sprout hips.

In my family, we ate all the sugary cereals—Fruit Loops, Trix, Lucky Charms—you name it, we ate it. Recently mentioned on the news, they have linked the food dyes from these sugary cereals listed above to the dreaded rise in autism. But now I don't even bring those cereals into the house. The worst it gets is Cheerios or Kix.

My daughter is fully aware of her limits, so she is thrilled to get even the slightest treat, like fruit rolls from farmers market or yogurt stars from Trader Joes. She will even tell me sometimes her tummy hurts from eating too much sugar. I also don't mind treating her to the KIND bars that have dark chocolate and only 5 grams of sugar. The nuts are good protein. What she loves most are by Dr. Schulze – the Original Superfood bars.

One of the Venice Moms with a Ph.D. helped me when Mario and I had arguments about sugar. When it comes to men, they need facts and figures. She came to my rescue with this helpful information:

"Sugar is added to over 80% of the foods in the grocery store. This added sugar is not the pure unadulterated cane sugar that our ancestors ate either. The most commonly added sugar is high fructose corn syrup which is an industrial food product and is not a natural occurring substance and is not processed in the body in the same way as cane sugar. In fact, because of how it is produced it requires no digestion and so is rapidly absorbed into the blood stream going directly to the liver causing liver damage and metabolic disturbances. In addition to HFCS, any type of sugar we are consuming today is highly

processed, devoid of all nutrients and in fact depletes the body of nutrients. Excess sugar depresses immunity in children and causes a

50% drop in the ability of their cells to engulf bacteria and germs. Children are much more sensitive to sugar and the glucose spikes associated with sugar ingestion which have been shown to decrease learning performance and cause more hyperactivity. Two hundred years ago, the average American ate two pounds of sugar a year. Today, the average child consumes 135 pounds a year. Along with this increase is a 30% increase in type 2 diabetes among children. Sugar is not harmless and it is as bad as they say. Do your research - sugar is about as bad as it gets."

-Tiffany Wright, Ph.D., The LA Skinny Coach

Letting it All Go

The more women keep trying to stay young and alter their faces or bodies, the more men seem to be interested in women who are more authentic, more natural and less plastic. Recently, I was informed that a woman with my breast type was far more attractive than my perky silicone counterparts and that women now pay thousands more dollars for the teardrop shape implants so they will look more natural.

I always thought it was the contrary. I was always flattered if someone asked me if my boobs were fake. Of course, that doesn't happen unless I'm wearing a bra. Oddly, in the face of genetics, I never had perky boobs even for a minute. They came in naturally saggy. Weird, if you consider I had been wearing a training bra since the 6th grade. I didn't sprout boobs until I was almost 15.

As you might imagine, now that I've had a late pregnancy and nursed my baby for 18 months, my breasts hang so low that if I bend my elbows at a 90-degree angle and point my fingers straight in front of me, my nipples hang only about an inch or two above my forearms. It's a scary sight. My boobs may as well be in a national geographic photo spread. The good news is, since nursing, I've permanently grown a full cup size and if I wear a bra, it would *appear* that I have a great rack!

One of the horrors of pregnancy is what happens to your nipples. They expand in diameter and become darker. Mine were almost a dark shade of brownish purple. They have since reverted to their natural size and pinkish hue, but that is definitely a bizarre sight when you witness it on your own body.

There is basically a laundry list of unsightly changes that happen during pregnancy and make you feel like your body has become one big science experiment. A nice little supplement to the nipple magnification—the weird random skin tags that appear around your neck. I was assured they would fall away after pregnancy, and I am happy to tell you, the skin tags have left the body!

Speaking of letting it all go… putting this information on the page is actually making me feel even more naked and vulnerable than childbirth did. Having children can sometimes help you let go of all control and just lay it all out there. Mario's best pal Ivor recently tried to ask me when I was going to have my book published. Instead he uttered, "When are you going to have your bush publicked?" I think he has that one right. *It's* officially *public!*

New Priorities

Once you have your precious bundle, your priorities change so much and you are exhausted. Nature has its way of helping you *not* care as much about the superficial things we hold on to, like our vanity. I always thought I would definitely want sex or certainly care about my looks after having a baby. What single woman doesn't think those same thoughts? Trust me — it changes.

I did have a sex drive during the pregnancy, even with the discomfort as the birth came closer. Surprisingly, many men are afraid to have sex with their pregnant mates, but the oxytocin production is GOOD for mom *and* the baby. They should get it while they *can!*

Obviously, once you have a child to chase around, you have a lot less interest in sex and a lot less time to look in the mirror and gawk at your flaws. You will have much bigger fish to fry. Luckily, you can't be nearly as sedentary as you can be if you don't have children. You won't even have as much time to shovel food down your throat. But don't fret! As time goes on, it does seem to get easier as the children grow older.

Losing my baby weight wasn't hard in the long run, but it is hard in the short run if you obsess about it. Unless you can have liposuction, a tummy tuck, are a maniac at the gym or have the discipline and determination to get a flat tummy, you may always struggle with your muffin top after your belly stretches out.

My girlfriend who worked at Cedars Sanai Hospital told me that the number one procedure there is a C-section/Tummy tuck. Is this any surprise? It *is* Hollywood, after all. In New York they call that a "Designer Birth," where you actually schedule it so you can choose the day of your baby's birth. But sadly they are scheduling a major surgery that may not be necessary and can actually affect their child's health.

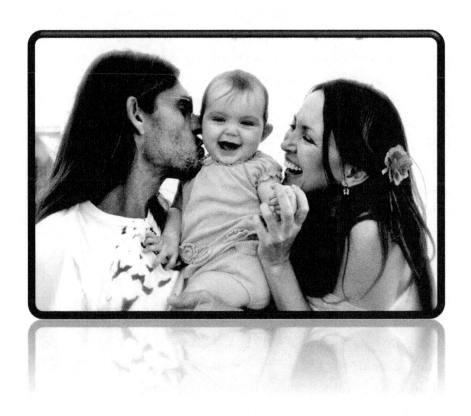

Happy. Healthy. Loved.
Photo by Annie Flatley

To V or Not To V

That is the question... I'm not talking about the obvious V word—Vagina, or my favorite—Vacation! One of the hardest times you will have as a new parent is sorting through all of the propaganda for and against vaccinations. It's very difficult to know who or what to trust, and even in Los Angeles, with the plethora of natural doctors, it's very challenging to find a pediatrician who will take your child as a patient if you elect not to vaccinate.

When Deja was just an infant, we educated ourselves and attended a seminar held by another local MD *and* a Homeopath, Dr. Lauren Feder. She just recently released a book *Natural Parenting*. Sadly, Dr. Feder has also recently passed away at 55, the same age my mother died, also from bone cancer.

What we learned at her seminar was that most illnesses that vaccines may (or may not prevent) can still be treated. That helped us finalize our decision. Perhaps because I'm inclined to choose the 'natural' option, we ultimately declined vaccinations. We agreed we would address these things only when necessary, if they ever came up.

We are acquainted with several chiropractors, acupuncturists, homeopaths and herbalists who all confirmed our gut instincts. None of them had ever vaccinated their children. Today their children are all in perfect health. One of my trusted health guru buddies in his late 50's, the son of two chiropractors, tells me he has never once been immunized.

I built Deja's immunity up as high as I could with breast milk and homeopathy, avoiding antibiotics unless absolutely necessary. In four years, Deja has only been given antibiotics twice in her life.

In fact, her immunity is so strong, that any time she has any sort of mild illness we take her to the Santa Monica Homeopathic Pharmacy. The Herbalists and Homeopaths on duty are more than generous with their time, providing free consultations and always succeed in supplying us with effective remedies. We have noticed very quick results with homeopathy. The best part is they all taste like sugar pills, so she *never* has a problem taking any medicine we hand her.

My 'friendly neighborhood mad scientist' Gunnar Keel is behind an amazing product called ViRxal. It helps improve infections and viruses — even herpes, shingles and HIV. I give my daughter half a capsule and stir it into a natural chocolate spread so she will eat it eagerly. It seems to knock out any viral infection very quickly.

I also still give her *Quinton* to drink and she loves it because it is pure sea plasma and nothing more than salty water.

I found another helpful resource is the website of Dr. Jay Gordon, a natural doctor in Los Angeles famous for his views on nutrition and natural parenting.

When Deja was almost a year old, one chiropractor told us that he can recognize immediately in a young child's face whether or not they have been vaccinated. He said it was obvious we did not vaccinate because Deja didn't have a blank stare. Since her debut, she has always been bright-eyed, hyper-alert and hyper-aware, never missing a beat.

I have seen that 'blank stare' in some children. Although, in all honesty, I've also met very alert, bright-eyed intelligent toddlers who *have* been vaccinated.

On the other hand, Annie's sister Liza's first child was perfectly normal until she was about 3.5 years old. She has been highly autistic since about that time. Her family can only deduce the vaccinations may have been what changed her daughter. Now that she is a young woman nearing 30 years old, her autism has been — and still is — very challenging on the entire family.

Recently, I took Deja to the ER only because her doctor was not in the office yet and before taking her to school with anything contagious, I needed to see what these suspicious bumps were on her skin. As it turned out, they were merely bug bites.

When we were met with a very grumpy doctor, he proceeded to lecture me for not having given Deja a tetanus shot. He was very rude and condescending and as I left, I heard him tell an orderly what a stupid woman I was. It was terribly unprofessional.

My favorite homeopath from the Homeopathic Pharmacy said she comes up against that all the time, and at this point she just tells them to bring on all they have so they can get it out. Clearly, she has had to develop a thick skin to unwaveringly defend her personal beliefs.

My chiropractor told me about a woman he knew who vaccinated her daughter (with that vaccine in particular) that resulted in several ambulance trips to the ER, as it was causing severe seizures. He said he would *never* put those chemicals into his child. He added that $9 of every vaccine goes into a fund for litigation against lawsuits that stem from their side effects.

Ironically, while telling him my story, I got a call from Deja's preschool, that one of the children in her class was removed because she had chicken pox. What adds more mystery to the mix is that this child was actually vaccinated for chicken pox.

This may conflict greatly with your own views or opinions, and understandably may generate feelings of fear and anxiety. I totally get that. As I have said, I am not here to judge or condemn anyone else for their choices that work for them. I definitely don't want to instill fear. It is scary enough just sorting through this information and trying to comfortably make these decisions. I am merely relaying my experience by sharing information I received that has proven highly successful for *our* family.

When searching Google for information about vaccines, the first page is almost completely PRO driven, so if you want to find the CONS, you may have to dig. Where profit is at stake, always bear in mind, it's "big business." If you search for vaccine risks or dangers, you will find dozens of videos on YouTube alone.

"Midwife and Editor of Midwifery Today

My Anti-Vaccine Passion

Vaccines are my pet peeve in life. The only "SIDS" case I have had in my practice (20 yrs, 800 births) was a little boy named Sam. His Mom had him in hospital with no meds and no intervention. She was someone I judged to be "too conservative" for me to mention the risks of vaccines. Her baby had thrush at six weeks, so she took him to the doctor and he received an antifungal treatment for the thrush, then she drove to the public health clinic and he was given oral Polio and DPT shot. He never woke up for his 3:00 am feed . . . . . I'll never forget getting the news he was dead. I told his Mom about my judgment of her and my cowardice to tell her about vaccine risks, and she slammed her fist into the kitchen wall. I promised her I would do everything I could to stop this health holocaust and to never let another client vaccinate without information about the risks. This is what drives my passion."

-Jan Tritten, Editor Midwifery Today Magazine

"Prevention is better than cure

... After these 4 initial cases I have treated more than 700 children whose immunity had been weakened by vaccinations, but all the time I kept thinking: We can't solve this problem with the help of therapy. The only solution is stopping vaccinations! I know we are talking about big business now, and that we are up against powerful forces. The vaccination industry is backed up world-wide by WHO in close co-operation with governments, financiers and industrialists. But this is no excuse for not starting doing something now. Because if we don't try to stop this madness now the coming generations will suffer not only from immuno-deficiency, but we'll see changes of genetic codes caused by the animal tissues injected into our children."

-     *Gunner Odom, MD (Vaccinetruth.org)*

Vacinfo.org says: *"EDUCATE before you VACCINATE."*

Some ingredients used in vaccines: MSG, antifreeze, formaldehyde, aluminum, glycerin, lead, cadmium, sulfates, yeast proteins, antibiotics, acetone, neomycin, streptomycin, mercury, monkey kidney, dog kidney, chick embryo, chicken egg, duck egg, calf serum, aborted fetal tissue, pig blood, horse blood, sheep blood, rabbit brain, guinea pig, cow heart, animal viruses, etc.

Whenever you go against the masses, you will be confronted with judgment. Medical doctors will almost always be inclined to recommend vaccinations. But when I read what ingredients go into them, I personally can't stomach the thought of it.

An article recently posted on vactruth.com included this information:

"In 1992, the Immunization Awareness Society (IAS) conducted a survey to examine the health of New Zealand's children. Unsurprisingly, the results of their study indicated that unvaccinated children were far healthier than vaccinated children."

1992 was over 20 years ago, but our country is still pushing us to vaccinate. Even recently with the measles outbreak, Mario has asked me if I want to reconsider vaccinating for this in particular. I do not wish to reconsider and I am very passionate about not letting the media or the government bully me into making any health choices for my child.

However, Mario's question led me to find Dr. Murray Clarke of Santa Monica who is a homeopath, a naturopath and a licensed acupuncturist. He has a book you may find helpful called *Natural Baby-Healthy Child, Alternative Health Care Solutions.* When I called, his very friendly receptionist told me several things I can do to boost her immunity which include probiotics, vitamin C, vitamin D and colostrum. I look forward to meeting him in the near future.

I have recently been reading *The Vaccine Book* by Dr. Robert Sears, which is extremely informative for any concerned parent who wants to do his or her due diligence. As a self-proclaimed 'pro-vaccine doctor,' he gives you both sides of the argument, and I feel he diplomatically lays out how serious each of the diseases are, how rare, and how treatable. He does believe vaccines offer more protection to those who are not breastfed.

Conscious Parenting

Navigating through parenting—when things don't make sense to an adult mind—can be so tricky. When a broken cracker sends a toddler into a flailing tantrum, we don't automatically know the best way to respond. It takes practice and constant awareness of their emotions as well as consistent reflection of our own agendas and emotional makeup.

I am learning that our children truly are our gurus and parenting is an epic opportunity to understand what our own issues are and how to not only heal them, but to rise above them. None of us want to pass on what we don't like about ourselves. Our children are, in fact, absorbing everything they see us say and do and can't help but become a combination of our best and worst qualities. I hate that becoming a parent automatically makes you a hypocrite. But again, this is my opportunity to improve myself.

I am so grateful to Barbara Olinger for the tips I learned at her parenting class for 2-4 year old children. She wrote a great little book called *Growing From The Roots*. I found it very helpful in my attempts to find more appropriate methods of discipline. Parenting theories have evolved considerably since we were children.

I wish I had earlier access to the information in *The Conscious Parent*. Oprah says she gives this book to every new parent she encounters. I recently saw Shefali Tsabary, PhD on *Oprah's Life Class* and fell in love with her outlook and approach. It could have really helped me when Deja was much younger, so I've decided to be happy I got this information *now* rather than later.

Liz Angeles

The following are several of my favorite excerpts from her best-selling book.

"Because children deserve parents who are conscious, don't we owe it to them to be transformed by them at least as much as we seek to transform them?" (Tsabary, 2010, p.14)

"As parents, we are often forced to react to our children with blinding speed, following our gut instincts, often not pausing for reflection before choosing our response. Before we know it, we have escalated a particular dynamic and within no time find ourselves caught in a negative equation with our children." (p.69)

"No one wins when we come from our unconscious reactive state. Emotional drama can only lead to suffering. So much of our pain is self-created. Unless we learn to break free from our negative interpretations, we will forever be mired in one destructive emotional pattern after another." (p.75)

"Our children can sense when we have a true deep respect for their opinions and choices. It's vital we recognize that, though they may only be little, they have a valid opinion that we respect and always take into consideration. As our children see that their presence is both meaningful and important to us, they learn to trust their inner voice." (p.82)

"If we look at life as a wise gentle guide, every circumstance is replete with opportunities to teach our children giving, receiving, humility, patience, courage, and love. We just have to be willing to identify these opportunities amid the grime. When we teach our children to find the emotional lesson behind every experience, we teach them to own their life with zest. No longer do they need to see themselves as victims. Instead, they are able to hold onto a sense of empowerment." (p.91)

"Life is here to be our teacher, our guide, and our spiritual partner. We are here to uncover our unconsciousness and integrate it. For this purpose, our past reappears in our present. Our ability to release ourselves from its shadows will determine how free our future will be." (p.92)

"When we match our emotional energy to theirs, they are assured we aren't preparing to strip them of their authenticity and in some way change them, which allows them to become receptive...Engaging in our children consciously enables us to issue an open invitation, welcoming them in such a manner that they can't help but feel they are being seen for who they are, free of our critique." (Tsabary, p.194)

"When my daughter speaks to me, I try hard to bring all my attention to her, listening with my heart as much as with my mind. I express respect for her voice and spirit, demonstrate reverence for her opinions if I don't agree with them, and remain in a state of receptive openness." (p.195)

"I tell my daughter, "I cannot take away your frustration, and neither do I want to. But I can be with you while you work through it."(p.248)

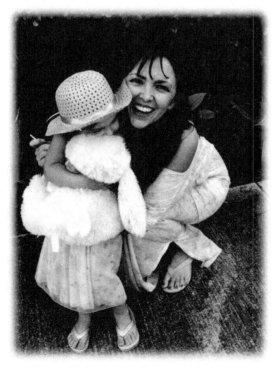

Easter Sunday 2013 – Bunny Day

The Best of Times

As a family, and as a couple, we have naturally been through our share of ups and downs. Some of my memories are just awful, while others are rather priceless.

After Deja arrived and I was able to ride a bike again, we got a low-rider bike with big ape-hanger handlebars. It felt amazing to stretch my arms up. I used the Ergo baby carrier (my favorite of all carriers) and strapped Deja on to me and rode it, while I was low enough to the ground that I knew I couldn't fall. Mario would skateboard behind us and she would always fall asleep on me. Those were precious magical moments.

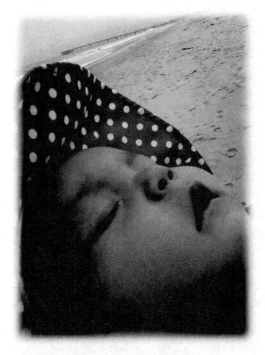

Sleeping Beach Baby

Mario always knew how to entertain Deja. He could practically swing her around the room by her pajamas and have us all in stitches. He was very innovative. He would do things like line the back of his pickup with a tarp and fill it with water to create a refreshing "ghetto pool" to beat the heat. He would also take her bassinet from her stroller and attach it with a bungee cord around a boogie board and take her sledding in the sand. She *loved* it!

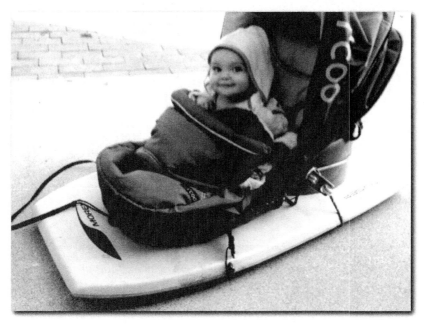

Boogie Board Bassinet

I am so grateful to have found my child a father who is hands-on and loves to keep her laughing and have fun on a constant basis. Childhood is so fleeting. It *should* be as joyous as possible. As much as money would come in handy, I have learned that the qualities Mario has in abundance are what will matter most to a child and be remembered more — by her *and* by me.

My favorite thing about motherhood

is having the right to

smother my child with affection.

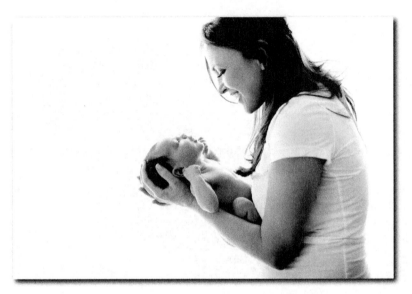

'Deja New' Coos at her Mama – Lori Dorman Photography

I can't stop kissing her. She can't stop me. No one can stop me. Knowing that is good for her makes it that much more freeing. I have had those urges with other children in my life, but they were never *my* children, so I always felt like I didn't have that right.

One of my favorite memories was when I was lying in bed with Deja who was 20 months old. She spontaneously decided to lean over and smother me with kisses. Ahhhhhh. There is no sweeter nectar in life!

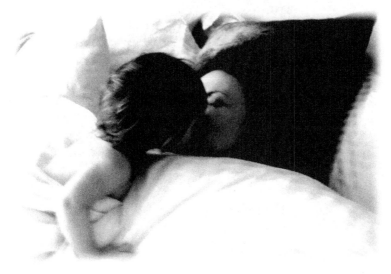

Deja Kisses Mama

Now that she constantly asks me to rub her (as softly as possible) occasionally, she will reciprocate and it is pure heaven.

One of my proudest moments as a mom was when Deja was around two years old. One of the girls who worked at the Kids Club at Spectrum Club told me how *loving* she was. She told me Deja would just slide up next to her and nuzzle against her and that if any child was crying for their mommy, she would always comfort them and tell them, "Don't worry. Mommies always come back!"

As she was telling me this, I spotted Deja kissing a little baby girl on her head.

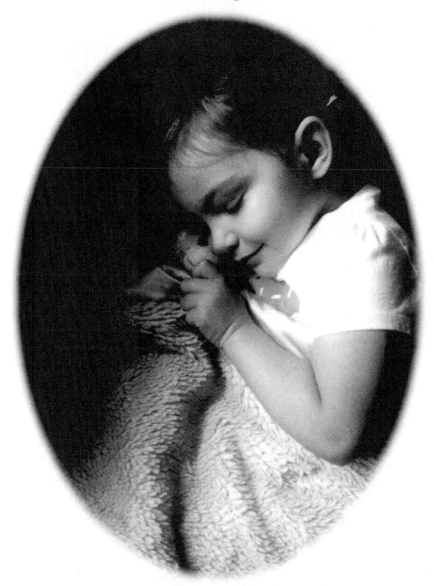

With Stuffed Monkey "Mikito"

Deja is so precocious and talkative that we were invited to audition for the *Jimmy Kimmel Show* as well as *Bet on Your Baby*, both on ABC. It's fun to do things like that, but I don't like to push her to be "on" for anyone. I figure that will all come in due time, as she is a natural born ham like her mother.

This was made evident to me when her transition class took a field trip to Giggles and Hugs at the Century City Mall. There was a child singing the ABC song on a microphone. As Deja was watching her, I could see her wheels turning thinking "*I can do that!*" (Perhaps that should be the title of this book?) She was only 27 months old, and was next on the chair and proceeded to sing the whole song in perfect pitch on a microphone, publicly, flawlessly and fearlessly.

Another clue Deja might be musical came one evening when our young male neighbors below us had a party with a very loud live punk rock band. Deja was in there on Mario's shoulders rocking out and loving it!

After that night we decided we should let her explore her interest in music at Toddle Tunes on Westwood Boulevard. It's a great program for the little ones. They expose the kids to all kinds of instruments and end the class with bubbles—their favorite thing. I highly recommend it.

The cutest thing that's happening is watching Deja learn, memorize and sing all the songs from the movie *Frozen*. But my latest favorite is her mimicking our silly foreign accents.

We recently got her into a classical ballet class in Venice and we *love* her teacher. MissMaries.net. The first time we went to Santa Monica School of Dance and Music, her ballet class also included tap. It was just the cutest, most precious time.

When Deja had turned six months old, she finally met her big sister, Adelina, who moved back in with us. It was really great to have her back. A healing had taken place between Adelina and her dad and it was wonderful. Best of all, Deja had a new BFF. They were amazing together.

Jasmine and Deja are also very close. It's funny how two teenagers who couldn't have been less interested in our pregnancy both fell in love with this little creature. She is like the glue that keeps bringing the family together.

It was about that time that the house became a bit crowded as Jasmine turned 18. Mario and Jasmine share the same birthday. As Geminis, they have a lot in common and tend to butt heads and press each other's buttons.

Just before Jasmine's 18th birthday, I had *just* finished creating a lovely lounge on our huge deck with the ocean view that included a massage cabana with a beautiful rug, Buddha fountain, amber lights, plants, flowers, candles. It was wonderful.

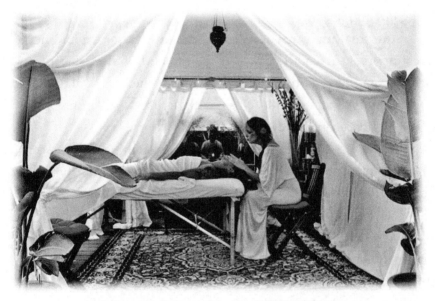

Massage Cabana, Marina Del Rey, 2011

On her birthday, I came home to Jasmine and her friends playing loud music, drinking, throwing water balloons, the whole deck was wet, and my outdoor sanctuary was a mess. I wanted to scream. Instead, I was speechless. So I locked myself in my room and nursed my baby. Nursing always swept me away to a place of peace.

Not long after that, the emotional temperature in the house reached epic proportions and it was then Jasmine's turn to leave home. So again, each girl left in the house now had her own room. Jasmine was highly resourceful and has so many friends and job skills, she survived like the independent young woman she is. In fact, she has had so much babysitting experience that she has now become a world-traveling nanny. As in most households with teenage girls, there was never a dull moment. Throw a baby in the mix and it's chaos!

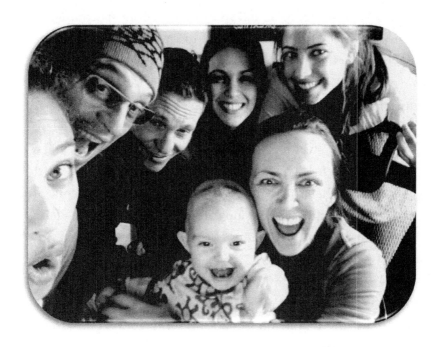

Adelina, Mario, Sergio, Jasmine, Emilie, Me, Deja
Head Shaving Day – One Year Old

The Worst of Times

Delivering a baby is hard, probably to prepare you for a lifetime of the 'hardship.' One of the biggest challenges of parenting is not having help around and everything is on *you* for that child to survive. I always wondered how single moms got through the day. What do they do if they have a sick kid but have to work? What if *the mother* is sick? How does any parent take care of a sick child when they are sick and have *no* help?

These questions plagued me long before becoming a mother myself. My biggest challenge to date: Looking after a toddler who is wreaking havoc in your home if your partner is at work or not in the picture at all, and you are in bed with the flu. That, my friends, may be one of the greatest challenges in life.

Those nights when your child is up sick and you haven't slept and you are stumbling through the house, trying to be strong... *fuhgettaboutit!* This is what you would call the *brutal* part of motherhood. What must be even harder is what parents of children with disabilities or serious illnesses endure on a daily basis. My heart goes out to them, for they are the *true* heroes of the world.

When Deja had a mild cold at two years old, I had no choice but to take her with me to Whole Foods. It was a hot day and she was having a tantrum. I had thrown on a long sundress, which required no bra or underwear. . . Or so I thought.

During Deja's tantrum in the parking lot, I was trying to hold her as well as the bag of goods, while she was busy trying to rip my dress off—but I only have two hands. The wind was blowing my dress up, she was on the ground flailing and I was trying to pick her up off the ground without the whole parking lot seeing my privates. Tantrums can be so humiliating for the parents. One day at the park I took away a popsicle that was melting all over her and she screamed bloody murder, as if I had just killed a dog in front of her.

Another night while I was still nursing, I was particularly exhausted and had taken a sleep aid that had me in a deep comatose-like slumber. Deja was somewhere between 12-18 months old, and had a terrible fever so she was sleeping between us. I woke up at one point, noticing how hot she was. When I woke Mario up to tell him, he jumped as if there were an earthquake in progress and went to get the thermometer and a lukewarm washcloth. He tends to wake up and quickly jump into high alert mode. I am wired quite the opposite.

He then quickly instructed me (as he tended to do, as if I were his child) to go get her a bottle of cold water to drink. I mumbled, "I have a head rush," but all *he* heard was, "I have a head ache." He then yelled at me, "Are you kidding me?! This isn't about *you!*" I was truthfully dizzy and lightheaded and needing to move very slowly. Because it was the middle of the night, I needed to pee.

I have a very sensitive Vagus nerve, which I am told explains why I have always had a tendency to faint. When I jumped up too quickly and stumbled into the kitchen, because I moved faster than I was prepared to, I passed out naked on the kitchen floor and peed all over it.

Then I suddenly woke up to Mario screaming at me from the bedroom, so I got up and stumbled to the bathroom and passed out again on the hall floor. I peed all over the carpet there too.

Then Adelina woke up and found me passed out naked on the floor in the hall (thankfully face down). With Deja crying in the next room and Mario yelling, she thought we were being burgled and I was the first one to be whacked. When Mario heard Adelina asking, "Liz, are you okay?" he leapt into action and came to my rescue. True to Mario's nature, he felt terrible, and cleaned up my pee that was all over the house.

When you are a new mom, your partner and you are bound to have conflicting ideas about parenting, which can encompass an infinite number of topics, especially regarding discipline. If you are in the early stages of parenting and perhaps busy nursing, you may not be working, which can also create financial stress and added strain to your relationship.

Mario has been involved with the construction of many high-end homes for L.A.'s elite — those who expect only the best, like Madonna and Rita Moreno. Even Jaclyn Smith told him he kept the cleanest job site she had ever seen. But at that time, it didn't matter. Only a year after Deja was born, in 2011 the entire country was affected by the economy. Construction took an especially hard hit, so we had to let go of our awesome beach pad and head east — just to the other side of the 405.

If you have ever lived or know anyone who lives on the west side of Los Angeles, you may have heard people say they don't go east of Lincoln Boulevard — they are AWOL (Always West of Lincoln) or they would never live east of the 405. *We* were two of those people.

Because we found ourselves in quite a sticky spot, our best option at that time was an apartment literally *on* the 405. When I would seek directions from my phone, it would instruct me to "Continue heading north on the 405," so you see — we were really *that* close.

Here we went from the most intoxicating ionic breeze and listening to the ocean waves on a daily basis, directly to the inescapable noise from the busiest freeway in the world. On top of that, our perfectly healthy daughter would now be subjected to constant fumes and soot in the air.

If you are forced to downsize and move, having to do so with a toddler can pose additional challenges. It basically sucked. Having a teenager and a toddler in the house can create additional pressure, affecting the optimal happy home life. It was indeed a rough couple of years.

Towards the end, after several months of bickering and therapy, not long before Deja's 3rd birthday, we experienced our first separation. I was relieved to relocate back to Santa Monica in a building where I previously resided before relocating to Venice during the recession of 2008. Santa Monica is a mecca for health food, yoga, spirituality, natural healers and of course, massage. It was where I needed to live to attract the most clientele.

However, it was very hard on us, and probably the hardest on Deja. She had several screaming tantrums once she had to see us separately, and mostly on *my* watch. I think she was angry with me because I was the one who moved out.

Co-parenting separately gave us heavy hearts. It was very hard on me as well as Mario to see other families around town, who were still together or appeared happy.

As we have gotten to know other parents, we have learned that what Comedian Martin Lawrence says is true: "No one is immune to the trials and tribulations of life." It's always comforting to hear other parents' stories of separation and reconciliation. It helps us understand our own childhoods that much more. Things really are so much more complicated for adults than they are for children, and impossible to explain *completely*.

After six months apart, we reconciled, and thanks to some very talented therapists, things began to look up. Mario is amazing at owning his stuff and taking responsibility for his part in it. He wanted nothing more than to restore our family. I was very grateful for that.

As with any family, no one could predict our future or how our family dynamics would ultimately play out. We just knew we all loved each other. Mario and I loved to see Deja every day and *really* wanted to raise her together. We are so much happier together than apart, but certain things can't be undone and sometimes reconciliations just don't stick.

Jasmine and Adelina are now 21 and 19, living on their own. They are beautiful and strong women, each holding down jobs responsibly. Looking back on it now, we made it through those trying years relatively unscathed. Based on their upbringing, I will always be impressed by how well they have turned out. For many people, it's a lot worse. We survived. The best part is I got a lot of practice with teenage girls. Not that I was any good at dealing with it, but I gave it my best shot.

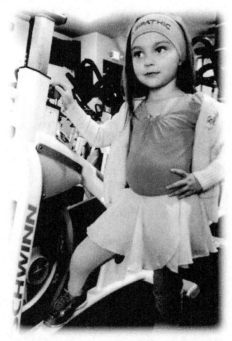

CyclePathic Fitness – Jasmine's Job and Passion

Deja Today

After our valiant efforts, our reconciliation did not stick--at least not *permanently.* Deja definitely wishes we were together, but she has far fewer tantrums than she did in our first separation. Yet even with all the drama, she still has a deep sense of who she is and a palpable knowing that she is safe and *very* loved.

She is a non-stop talker. It can be annoying, but it is often interesting and hilarious. Just the other day she asked me, "Mommy, if I'm not in your tummy anymore, why is your tummy still fat?" Nice, huh? A natural comedienne waiting to happen. But I wasn't laughing. She only heard crickets. Tough *womb.*

It never ceases to amaze me that she already has a stellar vocabulary and is also bilingual. We started our own YouTube channel called BilingualStorytimeLA if you would like to find stories narrated in both English and Spanish. I am very grateful to Mario that he will only speak Spanish to her. He gets annoyed that she won't speak it back to him and I just tell him to be patient because she is surrounded by English-speaking people. She will come around. In the meantime, she comprehends Spanish with no trouble at all and is even translating for me now.

I have been more concerned about having her around my friends and family who have potty mouths. I get upset because even Mario will inadvertently drop a few 'F' bombs here and there, and so will most of my best girlfriends! Annie gave me peace when she said, "Don't worry so much, Lizzy. She will mostly be emulating you, so if you don't swear, she probably won't either." I was in the habit of being very mindful of my words and dropping the profanity. I have since realized she is right! Now that I rarely swear, I find she doesn't either. In fact, she annoys all my friends with her constant policing of their language, "Hey! That's a bad word!"

These days, Deja is really enjoying her school, doing the monkey bars *all by herself* and all her friends and family. She is very close to her beautiful sisters, Jasmine and Adelina. They are all madly in love and it shows.

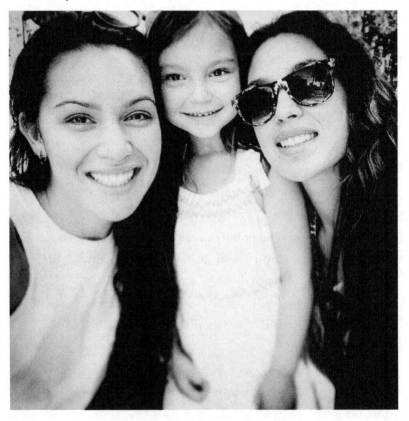

Las Tres Hermanas Hermosas

My Favorite Things

My least favorite thing about parenthood is there is really no way to avoid being what you always told yourself you would never become. It comes with the territory. It's impossible to set a perfect example, but to raise a child with the proper ethics, you find yourself becoming — the dreaded H word — a hypocrite!

So I try to make up for that by giving her the life skills that she will need and enjoy. Because she was a water baby, it seems only natural Deja should be swimming early on. For that reason, I recommend the folks behind SwimmingLA.com and the warm saline pool in which she was able to learn to swim. It's not only comforting to give her survival skills as early in life as possible, but it's a refreshing blast for her and for us, especially on scorching hot summer days.

I am eternally grateful for Dan the Man Gym in West LA and the gymnastics, trampolines, and toddler classes. This is where I discovered a program located there called Kids Artistic Sense. Sandra Caldwell who runs the program was brilliant with Deja. That transition class fulfilled its promise with flying colors — when it was time to begin preschool, she was thoroughly prepared.

We have been extremely grateful to Chalk Preschool of Venice for their compassionate teachers, excellent curriculum, long hours, and clean space. As I sat here writing in the sweltering heat of the summer months in Santa Monica, I was over the moon knowing she was in an air-conditioned preschool having fun with her friends, learning, growing and napping so mom can finish this book. Deja is constantly active, always wanting to play, draw, paint, explore, discover and read (or pretend to read). She likes to memorize what I read and then emulate her mom or her teachers.

More recently, our new favorite place on the planet we discovered is Garden of Angels in Santa Monica. This preschool teaches the kids everything from the basics to practical life skills. They learn yoga, dance, art, theater, music, geography, science, cooking, crafts, Spanish, sign language, and amazing field trips that teach them about things like sustainability and charity. The kids learn about famous artists and great minds like Picasso, Beethoven, Einstein, etc. It goes on and on. In my wildest imagination, I could not have dreamt of a more loving, well-rounded and idyllic place for her to explore and cultivate her ever-curious, spongy little brain.

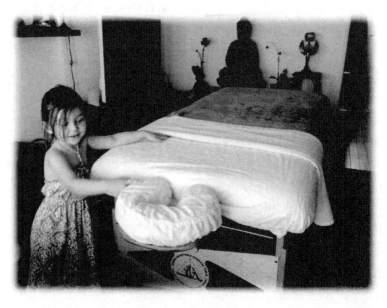

Ready to take over the family business?

10 Things I Wish I Had Known Sooner

If I were to give any other new mom advice, these are the ten things I have learned through experience that I wish someone had told me much sooner to save me time and grief:

Support Group – If you do not live in Los Angeles on the west side, you would not qualify to be in Venice Moms, but I strongly suggest seeking out a mothers support group. The e-mail list worked the best for me. It is highly accessible and *extremely* helpful. You can also find local mommy support groups on Facebook. Having access to this type of community support during pregnancy or during her first few months would have probably saved me a few gray hairs.

Clothing Swaps – I can't express strongly enough how handy this was for our family and how much money it must have saved us.

Mommy's Bliss – Gas drops you can find at Whole Foods. When your new baby has slept, eaten and has a clean diaper but is still fussy and screaming bloody murder, there is a good chance it's just gas. Another great technique that helps with their gas is gently pushing their knees to their chest. Bikram Yoga refers to it as the "wind removing" pose. Also, a new game changer called *The Windi* is now available at FridaBaby.com

Nose Frida – Those little booger suckers they give you at the hospital or in the baby kits don't really work. *The Nose Frida* is a siphon that you use to suck the baby's boogers out and it works like a DREAM so baby can sleep... and so can you! Don't worry - you cannot swallow them.

White Noise – This is a lifesaver when you need some peace and quiet. Your emotional connection to a new child makes their cries torture by nature. We got *The Sleep Sheep* and that worked like a dream. Until she was about 3 we used the Conch Shell selection on the White Noise Baby App from iTunes. If we were in the car and didn't have either option available, we searched on the radio dial for good clean static. 100.1 in LA. It would knock her right out.

Filing Block – I got so frustrated when Deja was scratching her fragile new face. Sadly, she was clearly annoyed by the mittens they give you to keep them from doing just that. I couldn't bear to clip her tiny little nails without fear of cutting her. The anxiety was overwhelming. Racha recommended one of those soft filing blocks. Their nails are so thin they don't need the heavy-duty nail files. It worked like a dream.

Nipple Guard – The nipple guard is your secret weapon if you want to get through breastfeeding. I can't recommend it highly enough. Every new nursing mommy should have one.

Harvey Karp's *Happiest Baby on the Block* — This book and/or video were so helpful, I wished I had gotten them sooner. I didn't learn that the first three months outside of the womb is considered the "fourth trimester" as babies have to come out while their heads can still fit through the birth canal. Sadly, I had *no idea how important swaddling was* until after Deja was three months old. It turns out, my swaddling blanket wasn't quite big enough to do it properly. A great new product that hit the market since Deja was born is the Swaddletee. It's brilliant!

Swing – A swing seems an obvious choice, but depending on where or how you live, you may be pressed for space, and you might opt to wait on that. And then you might later regret it, like I did. One of the best ways to put your baby to sleep or calm them is with a swing. It's a very successful noise reducer--for mom and dad.

Baths – When your baby has a fever, trying to bring it down with
cold water feels like ice to them. Luke warm is the way to
go. I learned that the hard way. In general, baths are far
and away the best and fastest way to uplift your cranky
child's mood.

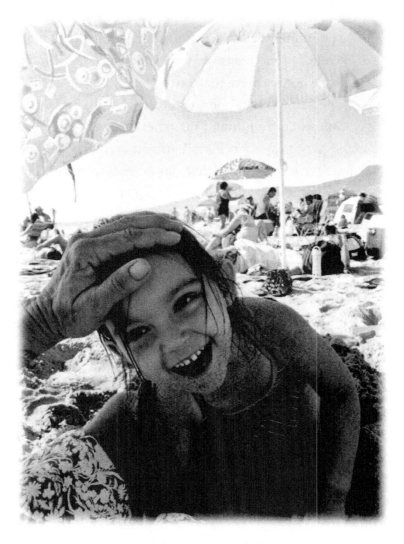

Epic Beach Day, Zuma 2014

Final Thoughts

If I had to do it all again, I *might* have another child if I were younger, had more energy, more money and could afford a nanny. I definitely know I wouldn't have a second child at this age. The entire time I was in labor, I kept asking "Whyyyyyyyyy does anyone do this more than once?"

They kept telling me "You forget." I knew *I* would never forget. But aside from that, I just knew that one child was *plenty* for me. I get to experience motherhood and all of its glories and challenges. I received my first hand-made piece of jewelry for Mother's Day. Deja made me a bracelet at school last year. It will always be dear to my heart. This year I got a necklace!

As I am completing the editing on this book, I realize I first started writing it at the same time Mario and I reconciled. Now as I am completing it, Mario are each settled in separate homes. It became very clear it's for the best that we do not live together. As much as we wanted it to work, we now know that it won't, and that we can never say we didn't give it our best shot.

I'm no psychologist, but in my line of work, people tend to pour their hearts out to me. If there is one thing I've learned from hundreds of conversations—with many who are children of divorce—it's this: If you know your relationship isn't going to work out early on, it appears to be much easier on children who are younger—in the long run. Even in my own family, I noticed that the older children become, the more traumatic the separation is on *them*.

We now have a deeper understanding and look forward to a life ahead raising Deja together *and* separately. Could we end up back together again? We teeter and totter like toddlers on the playground. For now, we reside separately, but are still united in our quest to cultivate for her as joyful an existence as possible.

Perhaps our destiny was to come together to create this special little being and learn about ourselves what we wouldn't have discovered otherwise. We do still love each other very much. Finding someone who understands you that deeply can take a lifetime. When you have children, you learn more than ever that nothing is in black and white and there are probably even *more* than fifty shades of grey. Either way, every day is a new adventure and I can't wait to see what tomorrow will bring.

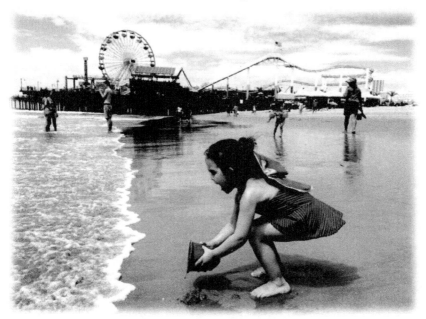

Santa Monica Pier, Summer 2014

If I had to leave you with anything, this is my greatest hope: If you want to become pregnant, trust in fate and relax. Enjoy your life knowing that all is unfolding just as it should. Try not to obsess. And above all else, NEVER beat yourself up--*especially* if your birth is not ideal. Just being a woman makes you AMAZING.

203

Whether your wish is to conceive over 40, have a home birth, a natural birth—whatever your choice—it is my hope that my story and my friends' success stories conceiving over 40 will give *you* additional hope. It is also my wish that you find in yourself your inner *belief* – that you *can*! Sometimes things just aren't possible until you *believe* they are.

Should you become pregnant, I recommend that you strongly consider enlisting the assistance of a midwife on your journey—no matter where or how you choose to deliver. And if she tells you it's time to go to the hospital, by all means, GO! Midwives have your back *and* your front. They make everything more comfortable, and the entire experience more meaningful, memorable and magical.

Acting as your guide and your witness,

midwives revere your birth in awe,

as the spectacular rite of passage that it is,

trusting in the natural order of things, and

hold paramount your right

to find in yourself

the empowered warrior

you are destined to become.

Special Thanks

Mario Ayala *for his loving support and being the best father ever.*

Annie Flatley *for cheerleading my every last victory.*

Racha Tahani Lawler *for being the best midwife possible.*

The Heathers *apprentices, for assisting in our magical birth.*

Sanctuary Birth Center *for their comfort, education and care.*

Ricki Lake and Abby Epstein *for The Business of Being Born*

Carol Song *for being the most delightful doula imaginable.*

Aleksandra Evanguelidi *for her wisdom and inspiration.*

Malia Hilliard *for her love, support and brilliant guidance.*

Linda West *for her inspiration, knowledge and encouragement.*

Heather Hayward *for insisting I write this book immediately.*

Venice Moms *for all of their wisdom, support and love.*

Alexia Salvatierra *for inadvertently introducing me to Mario.*

Asia and Devin Moses *for prodding Mario to impregnate me.*

Dana Haber, Sonia Azizian *and* Tracy Jones *for helping me get it together and stay afloat— through good times and bad.*

To our friends and family who loved and supported us through it all:

Michael and Patricia Schachtner, Paul and Tawni Heglmeier, Julia and Joel Pollak, Roland Jones, Audrey Hope, Gunnar Keel, Thoma Flatley-Griffin, Alexis Schutzer, Cheryl Lyman, Jan Plog, Jim and Mark Wilmarth, Dad and Liz Wilmarth, Jasmine Ayala, Adelina Ayala, Sergio Ayala, Susanna Ayala, Elizabeth Daggett, Angela Cerniglio, Carolyn Handling, Stephanie Weiss, Robin Stuart, Maureen Quinn, Jennifer Eagle, Deborah Cohen, Janene Schwan, Anna Richo-Moore, Ericka Danko, Sam Bayer, Alicia Fleer, Kathy McGurrin, Zoe Garaway, Josh Dembicer, Ira Josephs, Leah Simpson, Dana Lear, Jilleen Stelding, Jared Krause, Summer Forest, Christopher Gourlay, Ivor DeSilva, Sean Shirash Hattele, Dominic and Mendy Cerniglio, Michael and Zahava Zalben, Trish Loar, Price Marshall, Desiree Bartlett, and most importantly, my favorite person ever, without whom none of this would be possible - *my AMAZING Mother!*

Additional thanks to these fabulous local businesses:

Santa Monica Homeopathic Pharmacy, Laura Drago, LAc, Brandon Takahashi, D.C., Dan Bienenfeld, American Botanical Pharmacy, Costa Acupuncture, Exhale Venice, Two Bunch Palms, SwimmingLA.com, YogaGlo.com, Kids Artistic Sense, Dan the Man Gym, Chalk Preschool, Miss Marie's Ballet, Santa Monica School of Dance and Music, Toddle Tunes, Dr. Tony O'Donnell and Lori Dorman Photography.

I would love nothing more than to be a home-birth advocate and travel and speak publicly about my successfully 'Blizful' experience. Please write me with any questions, comments, concerns, etc.

I would be delighted to hear your personal conception and birth stories, most especially if you are over 40. Perhaps together we can share them with the women of the world who are desperately seeking guidance and hope.

Kindly visit 45andPregnant.com.

Facebook.com/liz.angeles
Twitter @lizangeles
Instagram – blizangeles
YouTube – LoveLizAngeles
LinkedIn – Liz Angeles

Recommended Links

BirthSanctuary.com

LACommunityBirth.com

LADoulaCare.com

TheBusinessofBeingBorn.com

PushedBirth.com

OriginalQuinton.com

BrightonBaby.com

DrFeder.com

DrJayGordon.com

DrMurrayClarke.com

NaturalBabyHealthyChild.com

VaccineTruth.org

Vacinfo.org

Vactruth.com

AskDrSears.com

ViRxal.com

Smhomeopathic.com

AnnieFlatley.com

LoriDorman.com

SkinnyCoach.com

MomTrainer.com

NiceNeedles.com

YourSourceForWellness.org

TakahashiChiropractic.com

DanBienenfeld.com

GadiBody.com

Yogaglo.com

Poweryoga.com

Swaddletee.com

FridaBaby.com

EZPZfun.com

BarbaraOlinger.info

AncientCurrent.com

CoconutResearchCenter.org

RadiantGreens.com

HerbDoc.com

DanTheManGym.com

KidsArtisticSense.org

ChalkPreschool.com

Garden-of-Angels.com

SwimmingLA.com

ToddleTunes.com

MissMaries.net

AChildAfter40.com

MothersOver40.com

LizAngeles.com

JustWhatYouKnead.com

45andPregnant.com

ABOUT THE AUTHOR

Born and raised in Healdsburg, California, Liz Angeles graduated high school with honors in Las Vegas and subsequently attended UNLV for several years. Self-employed most of her life, she has reinvented herself many times. For over a quarter of a century Liz has worked as massage therapist, often to many celebrities and has been featured on KTLA morning news and on Germany's Next Top Model.

A former writer for the Santa Monica Observer and editor for ABILITY Magazine, Liz is also a self-taught painter and has been licensed as a court reporter and Realtor in California and Nevada. Other occupations have included waitress, actress, model, promoter, sales rep and property manager.

Liz is currently a single mother living in Santa Monica who enjoys painting, yoga, hiking, biking, dancing, ping pong, traveling, shopping, massages, comedy, films, music, good books and most of all ... her wonderful daughter.

This is her first book.

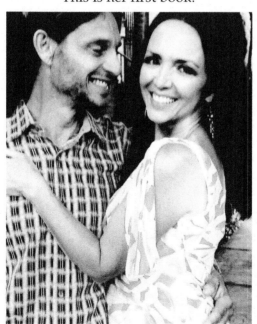

VISIT US AT
www.OnTheInsidePress.com

Where You'll Find

LINKS TO AUTHOR SITES
EXCERPTS FROM UPCOMING BOOKS
PREVIEWS OF NEW RELEASES
EXCLUSIVE AUTHOR INTERVIEWS

Join our mailing list for author
news updates and access to
free books and publications.

You can also get access to our
publishing requirements and guidelines.

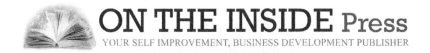

ON THE INSIDE Press
YOUR SELF IMPROVEMENT, BUSINESS DEVELOPMENT PUBLISHER

Printed in Great Britain
by Amazon

23389559R00126